Steve Miller is a successful moti[...]
company executives in positiv[...] ...developed his
inimitable approach – the Life Bitch method – when, trying to
lose weight a few years ago, he realised that you have to be tough
on yourself to get results.

His unique approach to self-motivation applies to more than
just losing weight; it is about gaining the strength of mind to
become the person you want to be, and realising that you can make
it happen. *Get Off Your Arse and Lose Weight* is the first of a series
of forthcoming titles by Steve Miller, in which he will show you
how to transform all aspects of your life – ranging from your work
life to your love life. It's time to let the Life Bitch help you make a
difference to you.

'The Gordon Ramsay of lifestyle gurus' *Daily Mirror*

'This should sort out men a treat' Barbara Ellen, *Observer*

'"Life Bitch" Steve Miller takes a no-nonsense approach to
losing the flab… Tough love, common sense and a dollop of
determination are his top flab-fighting methods' *Closer* magazine

'An old fashioned return to basics, a re-stiffening of the upper lip'
Birmingham Post

'Britain's toughest life coach' *Star on Sunday*

GET OFF YOUR ARSE & LOSE WEIGHT

STEVE MILLER

headline

First published in 2007
by HEADLINE PUBLISHING GROUP

First published in paperback in 2008
by HEADLINE PUBLISHING GROUP

2

Cataloguing in Publication Data is available from the British Library

ISBN 978 07553 1766 0

Typeset in Bell MT by Ben Cracknell Studios

Printed and bound in the UK by CPI MacKays, Chatham ME5 8TD

Headline's policy is to use papers that are natural, renewable and recyclable
products and made from wood grown in sustainable forests. The logging
and manufacturing processes are expected to conform to the environmental
regulations of the country of origin.

HEADLINE PUBLISHING GROUP
An Hachette Livre UK Company
338 Euston Road
London NW1 3BH

www.headline.co.uk

Acknowledgements

Amy and Ryan, my special niece and nephew, for lighting up my life; my mum and dad for providing a superb grounding in my life; Matt Rowlands, my agent, who has the patience of a saint; Eddie Bell for his fabulous support; Jean Wilde for fun, friendship and practical guidance; Brenda Colebourne – a stunning Life Bitch role model; Jacquie Pond for believing in me all the way along; Maggi Reilly for proving that even with a large family anything is possible with the Life Bitch; Alan Possart for his patience, love and support; Terry Brookes, my P.A. and soul mate; Debbie Fisher for the belly laughs and sparkly friendship we share; Jo Roberts-Miller for being such a quality publisher; Lindsey Gibson for her invigorating focus; my friends, clients and pets.

The Life Bitch series is dedicated to the memory of my inspiration and special friend June Linda Thompson, who sadly passed away in April 2007.

'Oh, darling, this is fabulous. I made it, and there isn't a day goes by when you are not in my thoughts.'

CONTENTS

Preface

Why I'm the Life Bitch (not a Tamworth pig)

Despite what you might think, especially when you've finished the book, I wasn't born a Life Bitch; it's something that's grown from within me. Unlike your expanding waistline, this is something I'm proud of, that's been in my head for years, that I have planned and nurtured.

I was born in a 'working-class' village called Kingsbury, near Tamworth in Warwickshire, but there's no Tamworth pig in me and I'll tell you why.

On the council estate where I grew up, people worked very hard, knowing that every penny counted, and we all understood that you did a hard day's work for a reasonable day's pay. It wasn't that long ago, but things have changed in our world and in my opinion not for the better. I'm not looking at 'my' world through rose-tinted glasses; I'm telling you why there weren't so many chubby folks and why people didn't come up with excuses – they just got on with making the best of their lives.

In our concrete council house there was my mum, dad, sister and me. Dad worked as an operative at an oil depot and Mum did cleaning jobs. They are both grafters and are only just coming up for retirement. They taught me to be ambitious and one of my core Life Bitch principles: you get out of life what you put in. This is a home truth that I hold dear to my heart and it is what drives me, in a very personal sense, on my Life Bitch crusade.

The biggest single influence on me when I was growing up was my mum, and it was from her that I got the values I cherish. When we were unsure of ourselves or messing around she would say, 'Don't faff about – just do it,' or 'Just get to the point.' You could say my mum's the original Life Bitch because she made me appreciate that an honest, no-nonsense attitude achieves results.

I've never forgotten the environment in which Mum's sound advice was given. The community had a real sense of unity, especially at Christmas, when we would be in and out of each other's houses, sharing hospitality. I grew up appreciating that the turkey on Christmas Day was a luxury and that my folks had worked hard to provide it. We saw things like a colour television as a massive treat. Things like this just weren't taken for granted, and we were grateful for the small things in life.

I learnt a lot from Mum, some of which comes into the book, particularly practical advice for weight control. For example, she used to say, 'Stop making silly excuses. If you want to lose weight, keep your trap shut.' Her view, and mine, is very much about using your common sense and not stuffing your face with food or resorting to fad diets and pills.

As I look back on the common-sense attitudes I grew up with, they are still incredibly relevant now because we have a society that is cushioned and pampered, where we skirt around the truth that fat people are fat because they are lazy and choose to be fat by eating too much.

So you will have gathered that I strongly believe that nowadays it is too easy for people to get fat and stay fat. When I was a kid, it was a huge luxury just to have a packet of chocolate biscuits in the cupboard, things like takeaways didn't exist and it was very rare that we went out for meals. These days, chocolate, crisps, fizzy drinks, pizzas, alcopops, ready-meals and all the other processed shit that you eat and drink are cheap, easy and everywhere. But, hold your horses there! Don't you dare use the cheapness and availability of processed food as an excuse for you being fat! It's you who is stuffing the cakes etc. down your throat, you who won't buy cheap, fresh, healthy food, and you who won't shift your lardy arse off the couch!

My mum and dad worked longer hours than most to guarantee we had enough money to buy decent food. The real issue for me is that they still found the time to prepare the food from scratch, make sure we ate as a family and provide a balanced diet. My parents inspired me and my siblings to take responsibility for our own eating habits and to maintain an ideal weight. Don't give me that work/life balance claptrap; it doesn't wash with me. How come my mum and dad could provide a stable home life, go out to work every day, putting in all those extra hours, and still provide good, natural, nutritious food for the family? The answer is simple: they made the time because they knew it was very important for our health and well-being.

The obvious truth is that people are now being conditioned to be lazy. Children learn to walk and then quickly learn to sit down in front of a computer or television for hours on end. Adults are too lazy to walk to the shops, and sometimes can't even be bothered to drive to them; instead they order from the internet and get the processed food and booze delivered to their doors.

I truly believe that people need to look in the mirror, give themselves a talking to and start to reverse the negative impact of our present society on weight issues. They have to make simple lifestyle changes and stop expecting the state to wrap them in cotton wool and make excuses for them. They need to learn about sensible eating and exercise. Our ancestors would fall about laughing at the state of us today, with some fat people moaning that the government isn't doing anything to help them. Just 30 or 40 years ago, people would never have got into the situation where they relied on junk food and cheap booze to keep them going.

As well as giving me my no-nonsense attitude and common sense when it comes to lifestyle and weight, my mum and dad planted the seeds in my mind that would drive my professional ambition and success.

I left school with few noteworthy qualifications, but realised from my parents' pep-talks that getting good exam results (and therefore making my own luck) would help me to develop a successful career. I knew they were right and so I went to college to take some exams and I thrived in that learning environment, where I was treated more like an adult. This motivated me to go on to Huddersfield Poly, where I gained a qualification in business, paving the way for a successful career in sales and marketing (the only time I ignored parental advice – they wanted me to go into insurance).

From a sales environment I went into the world of human resources (HR) and training. For some reason, I thought the right approach in HR was a 'touchy-feely' one, but how wrong I was. What I later found worked was honest, practical common sense, and that was another step up to becoming the Life Bitch I am now. That's why I hold business gods such as Sir Alan Sugar in the highest regard. They say it as it is, they expect results and get results. Believe me, our workplaces are not the right environments for tea and sympathy.

Looking at what motivated me to reach the top in my profession, I recognised I had a talent and flair for communication (I was a Butlins Redcoat for a while). But, at the same time, the breakdown and ending of a relationship that I really valued knocked my confidence to a degree that I started to suffer from panic attacks. I'd read about the benefits of clinical hypnosis in dealing with panic attacks and boosting self-confidence and decided to try it. Not only was clinical hypnosis my cure, it was my inspiration. It worked so well that I decided I had to pay for training to learn its techniques, which I could then pass on to other people. Quite simply, this was the best personal and professional training I have ever had.

I used self-hypnosis to affirm that I was a great, worthy product. It allowed me to recognise that the things we get from life, positive and negative, come from our own thoughts. The end result was that I became a senior business leader and had the confidence to go on to set up my own training business in 2003.

I started off running Steve Miller Training from my front room, and at first I suffered knockback after knockback, but my determination and self-belief were rock solid. I wasn't going to work for anyone else again.

I now run a highly successful training and development company and my personal clinical hypnosis practice has grown quickly. People responded to my direct style. I gave them a kick up the bum and demonstrated that they held the power to achieve their life goals. That's when the Life Bitch as you will come to know him was born.

I decided to write the Life Bitch on weight loss because, pardon the pun, it's a huge problem and being fat is something I dealt with myself. When I started my business I piled on extra pounds by drinking too much and stuffing myself – I was greedy. There were no excuses; it wasn't the anxiety of launching a business, it was my lack of self-control. I was fat for about two years and had a wardrobe full of clothes that I couldn't fit into. It got to the point where one day I looked at myself in the bathroom mirror and said to myself, 'Stop whinging. You don't need to diet. Use your common sense, use hypnosis to programme your mind, as you do with your clients. Get off your fat backside and do it.' And from that day on those thoughts became part of the Life Bitch. The Life Bitch thrives on a diet of common sense.

Plant the seeds of success in your mind, and don't give up. It might sound trite and obvious, but losing weight and becoming a Life Bitch is down to you and no one else. If you're still whining, put this book down and don't pick it up again till you're ready to make a commitment.

Bitching the fat

Now you understand that the Life Bitch comes from my disgust and impatience at society being protective of fat, lazy people, and that being a Life Bitch is just part of my character. Right now, you too can start to be a Life Bitch.

> Sit up and take note because together we are going to bitch the fat.

> Be warned, this book is not
> your typical self-help book — it's
> a kick-up-your-fat-arse book.

16

My book is for those people who want to lose weight. It's hard-hitting, straight-talking and to the point. It's certainly not for the faint-hearted, and while it's designed to help those flabby in body, it's not for the flabby-minded. So if you think that you will never lose weight, then you probably never will. To continue with the Life Bitch and be a successful slimmer with me you have to believe in yourself.

Believe me when I say that I'm on your side. Doing exactly what I ask you to do will help you slim down, get trim and, more than that, it will help you get what you want. Because, let's face it, fat people are often prejudged so they often don't get what they want out of life. Many people assume fat folks are lazy, undisciplined and don't create the right image. I certainly agree that they don't create the right image.

> **The most important thing for you to know and understand is that you don't have to be fat.**

It really is in your power to do something about it, especially with the help of your Life Bitch. Get it into your head now that you can and are going to lose weight and join me on the Life Bitch programme.

Doing what I suggest in this book will move you forward in your quest for the body beautiful, but before you take the first steps, I ask you to see your doctor and get a health check to find out what your ideal weight range is and also to ensure that you have no underlying medical conditions. If you have no medical condition that can prevent you from losing weight, then take on board what you read here. You have no excuse not to.

I know that there will be two types of reader of my book:

1 The 'flickers'. Those who simply flick through the pages and do nothing with my advice and so stay the losers they are.

2 The 'digesters'. These are the winners. They accept what I advise, digest the ideas (rather than too much food) and then follow through with positive action.

Are you still with me? Are you willing to give it a go? Then a word concerning diets before we start. The 'D' word is for people who are like big fat hamsters on a wheel. They are constantly grabbing at the next 'D', hoping it will fulfil their weight-loss dream. Personally, I never bother with a diet, as we often put the weight we have lost back on. What I suggest is a lifestyle change, a change which incorporates exciting, healthy eating. But you already know this. You know you need to eat healthy food and exercise appropriately to control your weight. That's why, in this book, it will be rare for me to refer to specific diets or rigid exercise regimes. I will mention food and exercise only in respect to common sense and conditioning your mind so that you will automatically eat healthily and exercise.

> Now you're in a position to let the Life Bitch into your life. From this moment, I will be your guide and mentor to a slimmer, trimmer, healthier you.

Fat in the frame

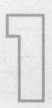

Why are we becoming fatties?

I often hear the complaint that no weight-loss plan really works. But none of us can ignore the obesity problem anymore; it's all over the media, from the very young children whose health is being put at risk to the grossly overweight adults who complain that no one will help them.

It's happening on a much larger scale than ever before because of the reasons we've already touched on. There are loads of excuses you can give for not being slim and healthy – cheap processed food always leaving you wanting more, using booze to prop up your emotions, lifestyles that leave no time to prepare proper food and the all-too-common attitude that life owes you something from the go – and these excuses are often blown way out of proportion by the media.

Life Bitch

> Let me tell you, if you do nothing in life, you will be nothing in life.

There are more fatties around now because people are not coping with life's pressures and are mistakenly stuffing themselves stupid and guzzling alcohol to feel some positive emotion. The secret to getting slim and being healthy is to take small steps to regain control and to start a lifestyle change. Now is the time to be thinking 'slimline'.

Is it okay to be fat?

It's okay to be fat as long as you remember that you're not going to live as long as your slim and healthy friends and relatives. It's okay to be fat unless you want to be able to lead a full, active life and play with your children and grandchildren.

It's okay to be fat, but remember it's the slim and healthy people who pay for your treatment when your health fails. Why should we pay for your lack of self-control?

But really, though, you know it's not okay to be fat when every time you look in the mirror someone you vaguely remember as being you when you were slim says, 'Let me out, you fat f****r. I've had enough.' Listen to your inner voice.

Real life

As a role model who admits her mistakes and as a person who has taken control of her issues with food and weight control, Sharon Osbourne takes a lot of beating. She's admitted that her weight has yo-yoed in the past and to the lure that junk food has had over her. She says that fat was something she cultivated while she worked for her father and had to do business with people who were older and tougher than her. She handled this by being big, loud and a bit of a bitch.

Sharon resorted to surgery some years ago to insert a gastric band which helped her to shed 125 pounds, but she's gone on to realise that weight gain and weight loss are down to her mind alone. This is what she said: 'It's something that we all need to learn to do, rather than try to rely on surgery, pills, shakes, and so on. I'm not condemning surgery as a last resort, but I know too many people who have had issues, be they medical or psychological, after having surgery.'

As a Life Bitch lesson, Sharon's journey shows that no matter who you are and what you've been through, there are no excuses for being fat. Yes, Sharon paid for her surgery and, yes, the same op is available to some on the NHS, but the fact is she, like me, has realised that the mind is mightier than the blade. You might have tried a quick-fix slimming solution yourself, and I bet you now know that weight loss through these methods is either an illusion or a temporary fix. What you need to do to become a Life Bitch is draw on the power of your mind to control your cravings and emotions. The day you acknowledge, as Sharon did, that it's your responsibility to lose weight in a sensible way is the day the Life Bitch in you is born.

Why you've got to be a role model

This is a no-brainer for me, and it should be for you. Why have we got pre-adolescent kids who are reaching body weights that are off the scales? I'll tell you why: because you and thousands like you are not being role models to them. If your children are overweight, and do not have legitimate medical problems, then it's a disgrace. A normal child who eats a balanced diet and plays and exercises should not be in that position. Not only are you handing them a poisoned chalice in terms of their health, but you are passing on all your unhealthy attitudes towards food and opening them up to emotional problems, such as the increased chance of being bullied at school. Shame on you.

It's so important that you get it in your head right now that you must and will be a weight-loss role model for yourself, your friends and children.

> Picture yourself as you really want to be.

No faking it

2

There are quick-fix solutions to appearing slimmer out there, ranging from diet pills and fat pants to even more drastic measures such as cosmetic surgery. Well forget them; you are not going to need them because they are for the weak and the lazy and they are short-term solutions.

These solutions don't require an ounce of effort, but usually cost plenty of money. How very typical of someone living a sedentary lifestyle to expect other people to do things for them. You are not going down these paths.

Fat-control pants

Bridget Jones's big pants made everyone laugh in the movie, but get real – how many people are actually going to be turned on by fat-control pants that they would expect their mother-in-law to be wearing? No, you need to be a Life Bitch and get the real deal by losing weight in a way you can be proud of and have long-term control over.

Wouldn't you rather be wearing sexy clothes and sexy underwear and have earned them through your own efforts rather than cheating? Imagine the feeling of walking into a bar, catching the eye of someone you find attractive and knowing you are the complete package, the real thing.

Cosmetic techniques

There has been loads of publicity in the last few years advocating cosmetic surgery as a means of getting rid of excess fat and trimming saggy bits. One of the most common techniques is liposuction, and if that is in your mind, I want it erased.

Let's consider liposuction for a few moments. It is a surgical procedure designed to remove fat deposits and shape the body. Fat is removed from under the skin with the use of vacuum-suction or an ultrasonic probe that breaks the fat into small pieces and then removes it via suction. If this thought isn't enough to put you off, then consider that you are risking your health instead of following a sensible weight-loss programme like the Life Bitch one.

Now, I can of course accept that sometimes, for urgent clinical reasons, this procedure has to be done to keep someone alive. But if this is not the case, if someone has surgery simply because they can't focus their mind and body to lose weight, they are simply tricking themselves. There is every chance that once the fat has been sucked out, they will continue with poor lifestyle and eating habits that will squeeze the fat back in. To think that liposuction is the answer is a bit naive and lazy, I would say. Do you honestly believe that when the fat is sucked out you will be able to go back to your old lifestyle and stay thin? I think not. So come on, pinch yourself (that should be easy) and get a grip on reality and your long-term future.

In my opinion taking the cosmetic route to rid yourself of your lard is a cheat's way out. You are really deluding yourself if you think that by sticking a knife in to scrape out the fat cells you will be slim forever. You need to work on the motivation and willpower techniques that the Life Bitch will instil in you.

If you have got the cheek to think that the NHS should pay for the treatment, think again. The NHS is busy enough treating people with legitimate, unavoidable health issues, so why should they spend time spooning away your fat when it is your own stupid fault you are the size you are?

Get this into your head right now: stop the visits to the fish and chip shop, quit eating greasy kebabs, and put an end to stuffing your gob full of rubbish. The real solution is to take note of the techniques described in this book to get your life back on track.

You should already know of the dangers of this type of surgery, such as infection, internal bleeding and other complications which, although rare, can cause potentially fatal breathing problems due to fluid in the lungs, severe allergic reactions and damage to the internal organs. And please don't think it's sensible to do it on the cheap abroad because you may end up in a world of hurt.

> I came across a scary report by Dr Frederick Grazer of Penn State University and Dr Rudolph de Jong of Thomas Jefferson Medical College. It says that in the year 2000, 917 plastic surgeons reported 95 deaths in over 496,000 liposuction surgeries. That means that there was one death per 5,224 operations. It could be you!

Hippocrates (460–370 BC), the 'Father of Medicine', said, 'The natural way is the only way.' He believed that the body must be treated as a whole, not just as individual parts, and that the root causes of problems must be treated (such as your lack of motivation and mental strength and the rubbish you're putting in your mouth) and not just symptoms.

Diet pills and potions

We've all come across adverts for them in the back of magazines and we are constantly being bombarded with junk emails about the latest superb diet pills and potions that will miraculously and with no physical or mental effort cause us to lose weight. What a load of bull. Very few, if any, of these magic slimming solutions are backed up by any scientific or medical evidence of note. These drugs claim to increase metabolic rates or act as appetite suppressants, but they can have some very alarming side effects if taken in the long term, ranging from headaches to elevated blood pressure and strokes. One of these is phentermine, a stimulant similar to an amphetamine, which was banned from being prescribed, but people have continued to pay hundreds of pounds for courses of treatment from internet sites. Some common side effects of this appetite suppressant are irregular heart rates, headaches and mood swings; if things go badly wrong, it's hallucinations and seizures.

> I understand that there are pressures on people to look thin and mimic the media darlings of our times, but, for goodness' sake, it's not worth risking your life.

I want to you start thinking about common-sense ways to lose weight. Use the Life Bitch programme and start with planning sensible, healthy eating and upping your physical activity. Not only will this save you money, it could save your life.

The 'D' word

Let me make one thing crystal clear: the Life Bitch is against you trying slimming 'diets' unless your GP has said you need to follow a special nutritional plan for medical reasons.

Consider that slimming diets have been around, in one bewildering form or another, for centuries – from cabbage soup diets to high-protein plans. The most common outcome, as most of you will have experienced, is some sudden, dramatic weight loss, followed by problems sticking to boring regimes and low energy, and finally a cave-in and a return to your bad habits and weight gain.

The Life Bitch message is simple and it's all common sense: you need to eat a balanced, healthy diet that does not overdose on any particular food group.

Follow the programme in this book and you'll see that you need to ditch the control pants, dodge the liposuction and keep off the diet pills. Instead you must:

! Eat as much fresh food – fruit, vegetables and meat – as possible instead of pre-prepared foods

! Make sure you eat regular meals: breakfast, lunch and a light dinner

! Satisfy cravings with healthy alternatives to high-fat, high-sugar processed snacks, such as carrot sticks, fruit, nuts and so on

! Drink plenty of water

! Avoid excessive amounts of alcohol

! Be realistic about your short- and long-term slimming goals

! Balance sensible eating with increased exercise – walking, climbing the stairs, playing with the kids, rediscovering sports or dancing

! Get off your arse and start looking after yourself!

I know there is a temptation to take short cuts in slimming, but that's as bad as giving up altogether and scoffing all the demon foods that have contributed to your saddlebags and double chin in the first place. Not only can the quick-fix routes be expensive and often as genuine as the miracle cures peddled by the snake-oil salesmen of the Wild West, they can be a fatal mistake for some.

Together with the Life Bitch, you will learn that the good things in life have to be earned through a little sweat and tears, but the rewards of doing it for yourself are huge. Come and join me; I will get you to your ideal target weight through a measured, results-driven programme that unlocks your barriers to weight loss.

It's time you took the time

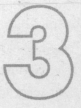

One of the lamest excuses not to do something about the way we look is not having enough time.

I was on a train once and overheard a fat lump opposite me whinging that he couldn't lose weight because he didn't have the time. As he sat there stuffing his gaping mug with a full fried breakfast accompanied by a few slices of toast on the side, I couldn't help passing along a few Life Bitch tips to this poor dumpling.

Unsurprisingly, he countered my offers of assistance and advice with yet another griping excuse. This time he claimed he worked 60 hours a week and it was impossible to eat well and to do any exercise at all. I sat there thinking to myself, 'Yes, I can well imagine him not even making an effort when "exercising" in the bedroom.' Blocking out these gross thoughts, I moved on and tucked into my fruit.

Life Bitch

The time issue is such a load of nonsense, especially when it comes to diet and exercise. Couldn't this guy have requested the fruit or muesli option for his breakfast on the train with no sweat and no effort? Could he not buy a pre-made salad and a couple of bottles of water at Euston station for his lunch? It has never been so bloody easy to be slim by choosing healthy prepared foods if you don't have the time to make them for yourself! Virtually all supermarkets and food stores cater for the health-conscious, for goodness' sake, and there is now a huge range of healthy sandwiches, snacks, smoothies and so on.

It is also a load of rubbish to say you haven't got time to do any physical activity other than dragging your arse out of bed and into the office. All you need to do is use your head and think about what you are doing each day. For example, get out of the office at lunchtime and go for a walk instead of sitting in front of the computer and chatting on Bebo, or take the stairs to the fifth floor rather than using the lift. Take time at the weekends to do something physical: take the dog for a long walk or go to the park with the kids and get active with them. It's easy to up your level of physical activity – all you need to do is stop being lazy.

So if you are one of these moaning doughnuts who pathetically harp on time and time again that it's hard to find the time to get slim, just get that idea right out of your head now. After reading the Life Bitch time-management tips below, there will be no excuse for not making time. So come on, let's get on with it!

Get hungry to manage your time

Too often we put little or no thought into how we use our time and quickly we get stressed. You need to develop a personal strategy to manage your time so that your life runs smoothly and you have time to eat sensibly, exercise and practise the Life Bitch techniques.

Imagine being able to fit into your life the time to get physical and go for walks, the time to read labels and check out what healthy foods are available at the supermarket, the time to practise my self-hypnosis techniques that will get your mind fit. Keep those thoughts in your mind and imagine yourself slimmer and more vital.

Get hungry, not for food
but to be a Life Bitch,
to manage your time so that
you can achieve your goals.

Prioritise your time

The key to prioritising is to eliminate what's not important and identify what's urgent. If it helps, try writing down the things that you have got to do on a Life Bitch chart and prioritise them by using colour coding. For example, use red for 'must do now', yellow for 'has to be done in the next few days' and green for 'can wait for a week or so'. Pin the chart to a wall and add to it as you need to. When you have achieved one of the priorities, make sure you cross it off. If you are one of those people that claim you don't even have time to prioritise, then get real and get a life. Start now and write down what you think your daily commitments are – looking after your kids from 7 a.m. until 8.30 a.m., your work commitments and anything else you know you must do each day. Take a look at what you have recorded and start to work out where you can slot in the gradual exercise I recommend, the time to go and buy the healthy food you know you should be eating and so on.

Just f*****g do it.

Use a 'To Do' list

A daily 'To Do' list may seem obvious, but it is very useful. Simply write down all the things you need to do on a particular day. Construct the daily list either last thing the evening before or first thing in the morning. You may combine a 'To Do' list with a calendar, or you may want to use a 'running' list which is continuously updated. Use whatever method works best for you.

Added to your 'To Do' list must now be Life Bitch items, such as '7 p.m. – walking' and '8 p.m. – planning a Life Bitch menu'. As you add Life Bitch items make sure you imagine the fat melting away because that is what they are going to do for you. Getting these actions clear in your mind will get you off to a brilliant start as a Life Bitch.

Avoid being a perfectionist

Some things need to be closer to perfect than others, but perfectionism and paying too much attention to detail can be a real pain in the arse when you want to get things done.

Who cares if your trainers don't quite match your tracksuit? As long as they are comfortable, safe and do the job they'll be fine. When it comes to starting to prepare your own healthy food, I don't expect you to be Raymond Blanc in the kitchen. Keep it simple, colourful and tasty.

You will find that you have time to get the details exactly how you want them once you have become more comfortable with the Life Bitch lifestyle; don't feel pressured to get everything just so from the word go.

Conquer procrastination

Procrastination, or putting things off because you can't be bothered to do them, is a real time-management sin. This is often the situation for people who want to lose weight, but don't take the first step to do something about it. Getting over this initial block can be a toughie, but just putting things off will not get them done or get you slimmer.

For you, this means getting off the couch, going on walks, throwing out the junk food and learning the Life Bitch techniques. But if you want to stay fat, then by all means do nothing.

Learn to say 'no'

'No' is such a small word, yet for many people it is a difficult thing to say. Focusing on what's important to you and your goal to shed the fat may help. You need to look hard at the time you have and prioritise the things you have got to do to be a Life Bitch. You have to win the battle in your mind and say 'no' to the couch potato temptations that have dogged your life to date.

It will be hard for you to say 'no' to friends who want you to go through the same safe routines – boozy Friday lunchtimes, drinks after work, going out for a meal and so on. Yes, do these things once in a while, but learn how to say 'no' too, and do something more constructive. Instead of following the pack, you could go out for that lunchtime walk and give the Friday night drinks a miss and go home to your family.

> You will feel empowered by saying 'no' to people and situations that are making you stay fat.

Making time for important, but often unscheduled, commitments such as family and friends can also help. But first you must be convinced that you and your priorities are important and that they don't just become an excuse for you not to lose weight. Once you are convinced that this is your life and that your goal to lose this weight is important to you, saying 'no' becomes a whole lot easier.

Flush the drains

Get out your mobile phone. Have a look at the names you have stored. In amongst the people who bring happiness to your life, and who are there to listen to you and give you their time, there may be some drains. These are the people who simply take your personal time but ignore your calls if there's nothing in it for them. I want you to delete them from your phonebook this minute. Flush away these little shits, they offer you nothing. It might sound a harsh step, but again this will empower you and make you feel you are valued. It will also give you more time you can use to be a Life Bitch slimming success.

Now you know that time is not your enemy and certainly not your excuse for being the king or queen of blubber. Go away and plan your days so that you can buy healthy foods and get your body moving regularly. Make time your own tool for success.

Getting motivated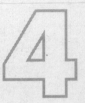

Personal motivation

At the heart of weight control we find personal motivation. Weight control doesn't just happen – it takes action, action, action. And it's the same for motivation; it doesn't just happen either, it needs a prod now and then. Personal motivation is vital, as it closes our escape hatches, our excuses for not getting to our ideal weight. And what a mixed bag of excuses we have! Here are a few of the most common, along with my suggestions for dealing with them. Take note, and let it be the last time you hear yourself saying them.

> ### 'HEALTHY FOOD IS NOT CONVENIENT'
>
> *No.* Many tasty, natural foods don't need any preparation and can be snacked on as they are, the minute you have a craving.

'EVERYONE DESERVES A TREAT NOW AND AGAIN'

Yes. But a treat doesn't have to be fattening. Why not treat yourself to your favourite exotic fruits or, even better, a non-food treat like going to the cinema (plain popcorn, no pick 'n' mix or nachos!) or some new clothes when you start to shed the pounds? It's important that you build your mental resolve by putting rewards in place, and the treats we are talking about are an essential part of the Life Bitch process.

'HEALTHY FOOD IS BORING'

No. It's a complete myth that healthy food is boring. Variety is the spice of life and there are plenty of healthy snacks and meals that are packed with colour and taste but lack the weighty calories. But how about starting the day with a homemade bowl of crunchy granola? Or a lunch of herb-crusted chicken fillet with a pine nut salad, followed by a dinner of Thai king prawns and wild rice with mandarin sorbet and lychees for dessert? There's nothing boring about that.

I can hear you saying that healthy food isn't satisfying and leaves you feeling hungry, but you can keep your body's energy needs topped up throughout the day with healthy snacks such as dried fruit, small portions of crunchy nuts and vegetable sticks. As well as satisfying your appetite during the day, they will cut down your cravings and tendency to overeat when you have your evening meal.

'I'LL START LOOKING AFTER MY HEALTH TOMORROW'

No. You and I both know that tomorrow never comes. Get off your fat arse right now, listen to my wake-up call and ditch the junk food.

Take Jim, who enjoyed a few pints a day and a curry accompanied by a couple of naan breads several times a week, which was often followed by his favourite chocolate roll with custard. At five feet six inches tall, Jim weighed in at 16 stone. Is it any wonder he died of coronary heart disease aged 55?

'FAT RUNS IN OUR FAMILY'

No. You're right about fat running, but only when it reaches melting point. Maybe your siblings or parents are fat, but that's because you're *all* eating too much! It's utter nonsense to accept that because they are fat and lazy then that's your preordained destiny. Show them the real you and prove to them that they could do it, too. Lose the weight you desperately want to by listening to the Life Bitch, not your friends and relatives.

'IT'S BECAUSE OF MY AGE'

No. It's not because of your age; it is because you feel some comfort in the status quo and in your eating habits and you are eating too much. Sure, your metabolism may have slowed down, but what you need to accept is that it's your lifestyle that has got to change, not your age. Take responsibility for it! There are many thousands of people in middle-age and beyond who have said enough is enough and have taken control of their weight – you can too.

My client Sandy was about to hit 40. She came to see me, worried that life was suddenly going to go off the rails as she hit this landmark age and was fat and frumpy. Telling the Life Bitch that the weight couldn't be shifted was one big mistake. My response was to tell her to get her fat arse off the chair so the poor chair could breathe, begin walking more and immediately kick out the laughable excuse that her fat couldn't be shifted because of her age. I spent time with Sandy explaining that there are plenty of people who have shed weight at 40 and beyond, often because they are faced with the stark choice of losing the beef or being ill or worse. She incorporated the Life Bitch programme into her life and eventually reduced her weight by three stone.

'WHAT'S THE POINT? I'VE TRIED TO LOSE WEIGHT BEFORE AND PUT IT ALL STRAIGHT BACK ON'

No. This might have been the case when you tried the latest fad diet, but remember that this time you're doing it the Life Bitch way and I do not accept failure. You need to start looking at yourself and the world in a different, more critical light. Accept that you are overweight and that you don't want to be anymore and, what's more, start to be disgusted by other people who are overweight. Now you will accept nothing less than success when it comes to managing your weight loss.

'I'VE GOT MORE IMPORTANT THINGS TO DO IN MY LIFE THAN LOSE WEIGHT'

No. Picture the next big party or social event you are attending and see yourself drawing comments of how great you look and what a change there has been in your appearance. Relish this thought and let it make weight loss the most important thing for you right now.

'I DON'T NEED TO EXERCISE BECAUSE MY HEART GETS LOADS OF EXERCISE CARRYING AROUND THIS WEIGHT'

No. This one is a real classic that I heard from a guy I'd guess was at least four stone overweight. This is just plain stupid, not to mention dangerous, because his heart was under so much extra strain it would probably lead to heart failure. The rest of his body would also give up the ghost and be prone to serious, long-term illnesses, ranging from diabetes to gall stones.

'I JUST CAN'T DO IT'

Yes. You *can* do it. I should know because I have done it myself and helped many others to do it. I do not have time for such a negative approach to life. I have had weight-control issues in the past and it wasn't until I totally convinced myself that I could take control of my weight that I actually did it.

You know you have a problem because you are reading this book and that's the first step in the right direction. So, yes, you can do it, with my motivation and inspiration.

From now on, I want you to reject all these excuses, and when you hear others opening these escape hatches, pity them. These people have chosen failure. Keep your own escape hatches firmly shut. You must not blame other people or challenging situations for you being overweight because it's solely down to you. What is blame? Take the 'b' off the word and it all becomes clear: 'lame'.

Willpower

Motivation acts as a springboard to launch our willpower, and willpower is something that we all need to succeed, especially when it comes to losing weight. You may be saying, 'I don't have any willpower.' Well, the fact is we all have it, and sparking your motivation will bring it out and make weight loss and weight control much easier. I will cover boosting your willpower using self-hypnosis techniques in more detail in chapter 6.

Above all else, do remember that motivation is your own responsibility, not anyone else's. So if you don't get motivated, if you decide to stay fat – fine, that's your choice. Don't then blame others or circumstances and don't look for scapegoats. You're the one who chooses your food and what you eat. You are an adult, so take responsibility for your own life right now. I can imagine some of you are already thinking that this is going to be too much like hard work, thinking that you'll not be able to stick with it. Well, stop it right now because I'm having none of that. Things are only hard work if you make them that way.

Ah, yes, I hear the excuses beginning again: 'No, but...yes, but...no, but...'

" Stop right there!
Don't get flabby in the mind
as well as the body! "

But how do you get motivated and bolster your willpower?

The good news is there are lots of things you can do to help yourself:

1 Draw a picture of your ideal body shape, making sure that this is realistic and healthy - no stick-thin, anorexic pics please. I want you to do this so you have a real representation of the shape you want to become, not that of some airbrushed supermodel from a glossy magazine. Keep it with you at all times and look at it in the morning when you get up, then four times throughout the day and once before you go to sleep, so that it becomes imprinted in your mind. Each time you look at this target body shape have a big smile on your face. Say, 'This is the me I'm going to become and I'm really, really excited about taking control and changing.' If you can't draw, just cut out a realistic body shape example from a magazine and keep it with you.

2 Select an item of clothing that you are dying to wear, that you would feel good in, that when you are able to wear, you will have achieved your ideal weight. Hang it up in a prominent position, where it is always visible, and keep it there until you fit into it. If you don't have something suitable in your wardrobe from a time when you were slimmer, use this as a good excuse to go shopping.

When you feel your willpower is weak, go to your room, look at this outfit and think to yourself, 'I can't wait to strut my stuff in this outfit. I will look gorgeous and people will look at me and know I'm a Life Bitch winner.'

Elaine, 33, is one of my clients. She found this idea particularly motivating. She kept her chosen dress hanging up in her bedroom for six months, during which time she shed three stone. She was excited and delighted to take this item of clothing with her on a holiday to Turkey. She sent me a text message from there, letting me know she was in the dress and feeling fabulous. She had gone from a size 16 to a size 12.

---

3 Write three — no more, no less — benefits of weight loss for each of the following areas:

✏️ HEALTH

e.g. more stamina in 'sexercise', healthier blood pressure, adding years to your life

✏️ PERSONAL

e.g. more success in dating, an increase in confidence, a balanced emotional state

✏️ WHAT YOU'LL BE ABLE TO DO THAT YOU CAN'T DO NOW

e.g. play with the kids without getting out of breath, say no to crappy food you don't want to eat, have more energy and enthusiasm for life.

Keep this list to hand at all times, so that when you are feeling some self-doubt or need a quick motivation boost you can read it and feel empowered by why you are doing things the Life Bitch way.

You can keep these thoughts and other tips and lists in a Life Bitch journal. Check out the sample journal on pages 254–6 and start one now.

4 Go to your food cupboards and remove any foods that are not conducive to weight control. You know the troublemakers: crisps, chocolate, biscuits and ready-meals. Take them to the waste bin and, literally, smash them into it. Don't give them away to others. You don't want them, you recognise that what you're getting rid of is unhealthy, so why would anyone else want them? This may be difficult if you can't bear to see waste, but it is part of your commitment process and lifestyle change, so just do it.

Enjoy throwing away the garbage comfort foods that are strangling your life. To help you along, I've drawn up a check list of some of the worst offenders (see page 261). Feel great as you throw the bad food away and prove to yourself that you are a winner.

There's no excuse, so get in there and chuck the fattening junk food out!

5 Surround yourself with 'radiators' and get those 'drains' out of your life. By 'radiators' I mean those who are supportive and want you to improve and be your best. They are brilliant to have around. Radiators are those who will say, 'You look great, but if you can lose weight, you will look stunning.' They are honest, encouraging and they will not give you false hope or be an emotional crutch.

A great radiator, whom we all know and sometimes hate but can identify with, is Simon Cowell of *X Factor* fame.

Simon is often criticised for 'putting people down', but if you listen to him carefully, the majority of his comments are designed not to hurt, but instead to encourage people to be the best they can.

The drains are like saboteurs who keep undermining your efforts. Take care: these guys are not always easy to spot. They may say things that sound supportive and comforting; they may tell you not to worry, that you're not that bad, that 'another slice of cake won't hurt' and that 'it's personality that counts'. But the drains are indirectly saying 'stay fat'. They think they are being your friends by encouraging you to enjoy the food with them. They are misguided and are doing you no favours, so ignore them and stick to your guns.

The archetypal drains are flushed out all the time in reality TV shows where people are vying to be the last man/woman standing and win public votes. They are the ones who go out of their way to be supportive to fellow contestants, but all the time they undermine them with meaningless encouragement and 'empathy'. Spend some time studying the drains in your favourite reality TV show and you will learn to spot the people who are sucking away your motivation in real life. Tell the drains to get lost.

6 Choose an affirmation that makes you feel good. Some examples are:

✓ I'm successfully shedding the pounds and it's exciting

✓ I am becoming more comfortable and confident with my new shape

✓ I'm in control and feeling more confident by the day as I melt the fat

✓ I am relaxed with who I am and enjoy every moment as a successful slimmer

Place it in your mind and let the thought of it become a healthy, everyday habit.

7 Walk tall from this moment on, knowing you already are a successful slimmer. You need this self-belief and confidence to bolster your willpower and defeat the unconscious mind that tells you to eat rubbish all the time.

If you're still in a rut, thinking that weight loss will never happen for you, give yourself a talking to, kick yourself up the rear and start putting some of my suggestions into practice right now.

The tips I have provided are easy to pick up and will boost your motivation in a variety of situations. Choose the one you think will work best for you and try it. Whenever you're feeling in the need for *more* motivation, try another. There's no shame in having an ideal dress hanging in your bedroom, a body-shape drawing by your computer or a list of three weight-loss benefits in your wallet. It's time to start taking your health and weight seriously, and to do so you will need to use all the motivation you can muster.

Motivating measures

Raising your motivation naturally leads to actions that will get you riding high on the Life Bitch programme. They are small, common-sense steps that will keep your motivation strong and get your body and mind going.

1   Walking tall: around your home, to work, walking the dog, walking up the stairs, in the park, to the shopping centre. Walk tall, smile and in your mind be aware that you are becoming trimmer every day. Let this help you to project your outer confidence. This will give you more willpower, boost your motivation and help you to shed weight as you get out and about more on foot.

2   Remember to police any 'victim' thoughts. If you become aware of excuses creeping into your mind, visualise a big stop sign. This might be when you've passed one of your favourite fast-food outlets and caught a whiff of something tasty, or one of the drains has dropped by again with a bag

of sweets. Each time, just flash that stop sign in your mind and take back control.

3 Combine healthy eating with moderate exercise and believe this is making you healthier and in all probability extending your life. You will be around longer for your partner, children, friends and family.

4 Ask a family member or friend to become your Life Bitch buddy and support and motivate you face to face and via text messages and emails.

5 Make a conscious effort to observe fat people. Notice how they often eat more than others – don't be sympathetic about it, let it repulse you. If their seemingly never ending hunger is not related to a medical condition, they should stop feeding their fat. Feel disgust and use that disgust for your own motivation to control your weight.

6 Start to leave food on your plate. Yes, I said leave food. If you start to leave food from the large portions you have become used to, you will soon enjoy the feeling of achievement that this gives you.

Forget all that rubbish about eating it all up because there are people starving in the world. You eating everything in sight isn't going to help feed them. If you're worried about world poverty and starvation then join a political group or make a donation to charity.

7 Eat slowly and be proud to admit it when you are full and want no more. Chewing your food slowly is important for several physical and psychological reasons. It is a natural way to eat less because the stomach will get around to telling your brain that it's full more quickly. Compare this to when you are wolfing down packets of chocolate biscuits or tucking away a Chinese takeaway – you always want more and don't ever feel your hunger is satisfied. Then suddenly, after you've gorged yourself, you feel stuffed and start to hate yourself and regret eating so much. So don't eat quickly. The slower chewing of your food will also help your digestive system and contribute to your overall sense of well-being. You might also think about cleaning your teeth after each meal, as this gives a further signal to the brain that you have eaten enough by clearing out your taste bud sensors which are encouraging you to eat more.

8 Treat yourself for having the motivation to control your weight, but not by going on an unhealthy binge. Instead buy yourself a new item of clothing or a beauty treatment, or, at no cost, have an extra long soak in the bath. Whatever floats your boat!

9 Keep imagining the feeling of ease and comfort when you wear clothes as a trim person, and how awkward and awful fat people feel when they try to squeeze into their clothes.

FACT Fat people often feel awkward, under-confident and uncomfortable when they try to squeeze into a favourite outfit. I know exactly how that feels. There was a time when I'd ballooned from a 30-inch waist to a 36. When I forced myself into a pair of 34-inch-waist trousers I looked like a question mark with my belly sticking out.

If this is your experience now, use it to your advantage.

Motivate your mind to experience the wonderful physical and psychological sensation as you slip into clothes that make you feel and look fantastic. Imagine this as a reality right now – good, isn't it? Think about this successful outcome on a daily basis. For me, it is the medicine the mind needs to be able to achieve great things.

We have gone through a host of tips to help you get motivated and actions that will help to keep your mind on track and your body up to the challenges. I want you to keep a Life Bitch journal and write down daily the actions you have taken to get motivated to achieve your ideal weight (see the sample journal on pages 254–6). This journal ritual is another effective tool that will help you programme your mind to achieve your ideal weight. Looking back on your progress and your successes will be a great motivator and will bolster your resolve to keep the weight off. Losers may start a journal but soon give it up. Be a winner – keep at it and you'll have something that you can dip into for inspiration and support when you need it.

So now you have no excuse. You have plenty of ways to help you become motivated to move from being a fatty to being a healthy, slim person.

All about attitude

Your attitude is going to play a big part in moving you forward to that ideal weight. With a positive attitude, you will find you are more driven, fulfilled and 100 per cent focused on becoming a successful Life Bitch weight-loss role model. Why do I say 100 per cent? This comes from breaking the word itself down into components. Attitude: let's take each letter and give it a score depending on where it falls in the alphabet.

A	=	1
T	=	20
T	=	20
I	=	9
T	=	20
U	=	21
D	=	4
E	=	5
TOTAL: 100		

Attitude is all about being 100 per cent committed, all of the time, to being slim, trim, fit and healthy. Anything less just won't do, so monitor your attitude at all times. Keep it positive because your weight outcome will ultimately be determined by it. Your attitude drives your behaviours, including, among other things, your eating habits, body language and the results you achieve in your life. A positive attitude will help you to carry out the actions described in this book, to understand why you are doing this and to be successful. A negative attitude automatically steers us away from achieving our goals. If you find yourself waking up one day with a negative attitude, give yourself one hell of a talking to, grow up, stop behaving like a child and turn it around immediately. Remember: attitude is a choice and it's yours. So don't try to tell me that others make you feel as you do so you can't lose weight. That is your choice. Accept it. I want a positive attitude from you.

Take the time to read one of my favourite pieces on attitude:

The longer I live, the more I realise the impact of attitude on life. Attitude, to me, is more important than facts. It is more important than the past, than education, than money, than circumstances, than failures, than successes, than what other people think or say or do. It is more important than appearance, giftedness or skill. It will make or break a company, a church, a home. The remarkable thing is we have a choice every day regarding the attitude we will embrace for that day. We cannot change our past, we cannot change the fact that people will act in a certain way. We cannot change the inevitable. The only thing we can do is play on the one string we have, and that is OUR ATTITUDE. I am convinced that life is 10 per cent what happens to me and 90 per cent how I react to it.

CHARLES SWINDOLL

Life Bitch

Real life

Margaret, a career woman who was a successful senior training professional, had a life-changing experience that needed Life Bitching. She was about to complete her senior professional qualifications in human resources when she had an encounter with a bus that resulted in a severe bang on the head and several weeks off work. Everything in her life changed there and then.

Margaret describes the impact on her confidence: 'The physical injuries healed, but what I hadn't anticipated was the impact to my emotional well-being. My confidence was at an all-time low, I suffered horrendous panic attacks and became daunted by the prospect of returning to work, not sure if I could cope.

'I felt safest at home and became an expert at eating junk food, loafing around and watching daytime TV, which compounded the destructive cycle I was in. As my weight ballooned, my confidence became even lower.'

After talking to me, Margaret realised that she had to do something and that perhaps the answer to her problems was within herself.

'To get back my self-esteem and control of my life, I followed a simple programme. Each day I would affirm positive thoughts and images to myself. I also looked for positive role models in celebrities and stars who maintain a healthy, attractive figure, and my mentor here was Kate Winslet.

'The techniques have helped inspire me to continue developing myself and achieving in both my personal and professional life. The ability to believe in myself and to mentally overcome barriers that were once placed in my mind has been life-changing.'

Here is a quick summary of my top tips to keep you on a path of motivation:

the
BITCH *list*

- Stop making excuses – just do it!
- Draw or get hold of a picture of your ideal body shape. Close your eyes and visualise yourself with this new shape.
- Hang your ideal outfit in a prominent place and look at it when you feel lacking in willpower.
- Write down the benefits of weight loss.
- Bin the junk food.
- Keep a Life Bitch journal – it will bolster your drive and motivation to lose weight.
- Block off the drains right now and surround yourself with radiators.
- Choose a positive affirmation and drum it into your mind.
- Walk everywhere you can, with your head held high.
- If you feel temptation or doubt, flash the big red stop sign in your mind.
- Find a Life Bitch buddy.
- Feel disgusted by the fat people surrounding you.

the BITCH *list*

- Eat your food slowly and enjoy each mouthful. It will leave you feeling full and satisfied more quickly than shovelling down heaps of rubbish. Leave food on your plate.
- Clean your teeth after meals.
- Plan and look forward to the rewards on your journey, whether it be buying clothes you never thought you could wear or wearing a bikini on your dream holiday.
- Be driven by your results, even if they are small – losing a little weight, clothes feeling slacker, the odd compliment.
- Always maintain a positive attitude.

Too stressed to weigh less?

5

For the majority of us, stress in life is unavoidable and is something we have to deal with. Stress can come from anything from managing a home and caring for children to being the outwardly confident CEO of a big company. We know it's there all around us and it's scary.

A Liverpool University study published in 2004 reported that women are six times more likely than men to overeat as a coping mechanism to deal with stress. There is a lot of truth in the saying that 'women are emotional beings'. When they become emotional for whatever reason they are likely to channel this into a physical action such as shouting or eating. That means when there's an emotional overload they are likely to reach for the chocolate digestives. Men, on the other hand, are more likely to deal with stress by switching off their emotional responses and going with instincts that allow them to focus on the situation and avoid the emotional crutches.

As well as the academic evidence, I am aware from my own experiences and those of my clients that women are more likely to comfort eat than men. And nowadays they are also tending to binge drink much more as a stress response. It's a double whammy for women! This emotional eating is a natural way to deny negative feelings such as anxiety, sadness, guilt or jealousy.

One of the physical causes of emotional eating is an increased level of cortisol, the stress hormone, which can create cravings for food. It may also be caused by childhood conditioning. Parents often provide children with goodies such as ice creams or sweets to make up for difficult or challenging experiences. Some of us therefore grow up associating these foods with feeling better when faced with stress, and this can quickly spiral out of control.

Ask yourself this: are you one of those people that wants to reach for the biscuit tin, get hold of a chocolate bar, or treat yourself to a bag of chips or a takeaway when the stress kicks in?

If you are an emotional eater, it is time to get a grip and use the Life Bitch coping mechanisms. If your emotional problems are the result of a bereavement, divorce or depression, then visit your GP for additional advice and support. However, if you're simply moping about not getting that job you applied for, or the dream holiday you were unable to afford, then get over it!

Let go of this behaviour and accept that new responses have to take hold if you are to say bye-bye to food as an emotional feeder.

Practise relaxation

Each day practise a relaxation technique for around 15 minutes. This will help you to rebalance and bring yourself back to a sense of control. Simply find a warm, safe place where you will not be disturbed, sit in a comfortable seat and do the following:

1 Close your eyes and focus on your breathing.

2 Imagine a favourite place of relaxation, somewhere you know well or somewhere you have dreamt of.

3 Take yourself into your favourite place of relaxation, pay attention to any unnecessary nervous tension and let it melt away.

4 Imagine negative thoughts drifting out of your mind every time you breathe out.

5 As you breathe in, take in positive thoughts, such as being in control, calm, focused and relaxed.

Life Bitch

6 Enjoy the sensations of being so relaxed you feel as though you are soaking in a warm bath.

7 Finally, mentally count up from one to ten. Say to yourself that you will open your eyes at the count of seven and be fully awake at the count of ten. Tell yourself that you will awaken feeling refreshed, calm, focused and in control.

Make sure you practise this technique regularly, so that you can quickly get to grips with it and use it as a stress-buster.

Make up some Life Bitch treat troughs

Prepare Life Bitch goodies in small plastic bags – pop in some of your favourite healthy snacks. This is a great way to satisfy your grazing habit; when you feel stressed and tempted to eat, you can dig into one of these without getting into the vicious circle of stress, eating, guilt, stress and so on. Have these at hand at home and at work, so when times get tough you can get to them. It isn't difficult to prepare these daily. The secret is to vary them. Here are a couple of examples:

TROUGH 1

1 green apple
Orange slices
3 carrots
A low-fat yogurt
A packet of
   sunflower
   seeds

66

The Life Bitch troughs are a simple idea that will help beat the bad eating habits that stress can lead to. These are my common-sense ideas; use them as a guide to come up with your own. Keep them simple and true to the Life Bitch faith – so no chocolate-covered raisins!

TROUGH 2

Half a wholemeal
   sandwich of lean turkey
A handful of grapes
A small packet of
raisins
Organic orange juice
A wholemeal cereal bar

Bitch with your buddy!

It is good to talk, so get yourself a Life Bitch buddy. This should be someone who listens well, is comfortable with themselves and has time on their hands to give to you. Ideally, they will have maturity and life experience so that they can genuinely empathise with you.

Avoid the type of person who will treat you like a child and enjoy the power of moulding you. They will do your head in and offer little worthwhile support. Find someone who is going to inspire you when life is tough; that is the kind of strength you need.

It would be perfect if your Life Bitch buddy could be someone who wants to share the Life Bitch journey with you. Sharing this common experience will be valuable in bolstering each other's willpower and helping each other to overcome the challenges you will face.

Life Bitch

As you bitch about life with your buddy, let it all out, cry as much as you want and then agree on an action plan and follow it through together.

Go out for a walk/get a punch bag

Depending on your level of stress and your physical fitness, I recommend two simple ways to de-stress naturally that will also benefit your weight-loss goal: walking and punching.

If things really are getting too much for you to cope take a deep breath and have some 'me' time, whether you're at home or at work. As soon as you can get out, go and stretch your legs on a brisk walk. It will do you the world of good and you'll know it straightaway as you breathe the fresh air into your lungs.

It might seem radical, but using a punch bag or punch ball at home or at the gym is a fantastic de-stressor. Picture this: your boss has dragged your good name through the dirt for the umpteenth time and you want to scream and shout, but you can't. You know he or she is an idiot, but if you say anything you'll risk your job and you can't afford to lose it. Your normal solution would be to tuck into the biscuits and moan to your workmates. I don't want you to do that; instead save your frustration until you get to your punch bag. When you are there, picture his or her face barking at you and start jabbing away. You won't believe how good this will make you feel, and the sweat you will get going will be evidence of the brilliant workout you're having.

Among other things, the benefits of these quick fix de-stressors include a release of endorphins which helps provide a feel-good factor. They will calm you down and help focus your thoughts in a positive way. Think about the great things the rest of the day or tomorrow will bring.

This is all good stuff to help you let go of unhealthy emotions and of course keep trim. It may also be a good idea to walk or workout with your Life Bitch buddy so you can talk through your emotions at the same time.

Get it down in your Life Bitch journal

Write down your emotions in your Life Bitch journal. Express your feelings as fully as possible. Do this first thing in the morning and last thing at night to help you have both a good day and then a good night's sleep. If you wake up in the night with negative emotions going through your head, then write them down. This will release any negative thoughts brought out by stressful situations and help you work through the issues that are sticking in your mind. It will help to get these stress-driven problems into perspective and minimise the emotional responses that might be triggered by them. I want you to start doing this now because it's a simple, effective way to get stress into perspective and start handling it. No excuse – pen and journal now!

Another action to consider is to really let your thoughts out with a physical action. When you have got everything on paper, especially the anger you feel, rip up the piece of paper and flush it down the loo.

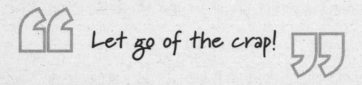

Learn something new

Finding a new hobby – something you have never done before, or at least not for a long time – not only takes your mind off things but also builds your confidence.

Something creative is often a good idea, such as painting, dance, writing or pottery, because each of these will help you to express your feelings and release pent-up anger and emotions. You will also meet new people and make friends. Pop into the local library and ask for information on local groups and societies. Alternatively, you may want to consider a course with the Open University or a distance-learning programme where you gain a recognised qualification.

If you are experiencing a lot of work-related stress then why not really get with the Life Bitch programme and change your life by picking up new qualifications? Remember my own Life Bitch story. By learning something new and getting more qualifications, your horizons will open up and you could get the job you've always wanted.

Real life

Take Tina, a 32-year-old professional who was dropping the pounds and reaching her own special goal. But having found out that her partner had had an affair just after they got married, Tina began piling back on the two stone she had struggled hard to lose.

Food became the crutch that propped up her emotions. Tina particularly struggled in the evening when she got home from work. She satisfied herself with junk food, including chocolate, pizza, crisps, ice cream and cakes. She would lie on the sofa with the duvet over her watching TV. As the weeks passed, Tina was beginning to return to the porky state that she really detested. As she became fatter, she also became more depressed.

At our first meeting I requested she visit her GP and clearance was given for her to work with me. Tina's situation was typical of that of many young women who use food to give their emotions a boost. We agreed that she needed to get a grip on her feelings if she was to lose weight as well as save her marriage. The first session was geared towards letting out the anger and grief she felt about her husband's affair. We worked out a plan of action to move Tina away from emotional eating. She did not want counselling as she had tried it before and achieved nothing. We agreed that Tina would join her local women's hockey team, as she had played hockey at university. She would practise relaxation and she accepted that she had to open a healthy dialogue with her husband. She agreed to mentally rehearse how she would talk with him; this was made easier by the fact that he really wanted to save his marriage.

Six months after beginning her Life Bitch plan, Tina had lost the weight and become stronger. What's more, she was also expecting her first child.

Get stressed less

For most people, it's virtually impossible never to experience stress, but the sensible thing to do is to identify where most of the stress in your life comes from and form strategies to minimise or avoid it.

I want you to write down in your Life Bitch journal what you believe is causing the most stress in your life and start to break down and examine each trigger in some detail. For example, it might be your job, so work out why it is stressful. Is it deadlines you find hard, a boss who's a shit, commuting? There are solutions to all these issues, ranging from managing your workload more efficiently to finding a new job where commuting isn't an issue and/or the bastard boss is left behind.

> Whatever you do, don't let food become your coping mechanism.

If you are overweight, you may have low self-confidence and low self-esteem and these factors make many situations that others take in their stride stressful – being in public, job interviews, dating and so on. Solution? Smile, because you have taken a huge step towards getting your weight down. The small steps we take together will help you to deal quickly with the common situations that you now find stressful. Key among them will be the self-affirmations such as 'I am going to be slimmer and trimmer' or 'I

Real life

Brian, a guy in his late 50s, worked with me a while ago. He had a goal: he wanted to walk his eldest daughter, Emily, down the aisle, but had put on several stone and was ashamed of his appearance.

Discussing how his work had impacted on his life, Brian explained that he was a facilities manager for a local authority and each day brought lists of other people's problems that he had to sort out. He wasn't coping well with the pressure and was drinking too much and eating his favourite steak and kidney pie with chips too often.

I asked Brian to write down the stress triggers in his life and together we worked on several coping strategies. He agreed to use my simple self-relaxation technique (see page 65) when things got tough at work and he also spoke to his manager about reducing his workload. These two factors had a quick impact on Brian's stress and he began to feel more confident and in control at work.

We looked at his lifestyle and eating habits to see if things could be improved and planned out a weekly routine that introduced de-stressing walks and sensible eating. We included a 'day-off' during the week, when he allowed himself some treats and a glass or two of wine, and he was even able to indulge in his beloved steak and kidney pie once a month.

The results have been fantastic for Brian. He dropped three inches from his waist, lost the jowls he had developed and, as Emily said at her wedding, he 'looked years younger'. A real health bonus was that the weight loss and reduction in stress lowered his blood pressure from dangerously high to normal.

The key to Brian's success was identifying his stress triggers and getting his work situation sorted so that he could feel confident and in control.

will be able to get into that business suit that makes me look and feel like a success.'

Getting stress resolved is vital to successful and maintained weight loss. On the face of it, yes, stress is a complicated issue which varies from individual to individual, but if you face up to it and break it down it can be, at the very least, reduced so that you can manage it.

Take some time with this chapter and make sure you understand why stress has contributed to your overeating because it's not an excuse I will tolerate anymore.

the
BITCH *list*

- Practise regular relaxation.
- Make up some Life Bitch troughs if you are likely to need a graze.
- When times are tough, turn to your bitch buddy for support.
- If you are feeling emotional, go out for a good walk or workout.
- Purge those negative feelings by jotting them down in your Life Bitch journal. If it helps, tear out the page, rip it up and flush the negativity out of your life!
- Do something new that makes you feel good.
- Sort out the source of the stress so that you can deal with it instead of constantly moaning about it.

Mind support: finding the willpower

6

Let's take a look at how you can apply self-hypnosis techniques to grow willpower and effectively reduce weight.

Drawing on the strength of will that's in your mind will make a huge difference to you. It's the difference between you being a lardarse and having a cute arse.

Where's your head at?

It's very important that you understand how your brain works, so that you can take control of the parts that will make your willpower into the strongest tool that will help you to lose weight and keep it off.

If your body has got fat, it's a sure thing that your mind has also allowed itself to get fat and sluggish. To get it fighting fit, understand the following practical advice and techniques and use them to your advantage.

Your mind is split into two parts: the conscious and the unconscious. The conscious mind is represented by your current awareness – your thoughts, feelings and here and now experiences.

The unconscious mind is represented by those of your memories and experiences that have been 'forgotten'. In other words, these memories and experiences are out of your conscious awareness, although they may well become conscious again under different circumstances. For example, as a child I ate some tomato sauce and suddenly vomited. Although that experience is done and dusted, is in the past and consigned to my unconscious mind, whenever I see or smell tomato sauce, I suddenly feel an uncomfortable sensation in my stomach.

The unconscious area of the brain that controls and influences our life patterns, memories, habits, emotions and automatic functions is also known as the limbic system.

Mind over platter

Getting your unconscious mind to stop telling you to stuff your mouth with crisps and takeaways is the key to getting the thunder off your thighs.

We are going to programme the unconscious mind to create some healthy habits that will slim your body and keep it that way.

In other words, I will show you how to achieve and maintain a healthy weight through habit. This will take your weight loss forward quickly because your mind will be programmed to automatically move towards the ideal shape.

Your bad eating habits, such as piling your plate high and craving high-fat, high-sugar foods, have become a conditioned reflex. I'm going to help you change that so your unconscious mind kicks out the cravings for junk and replaces them with sensible eating habits.

The techniques

In order to set up and boost your willpower, you first need to turn off the unhelpful impulses to eat garbage foods and eat too much. To do this, you must tap into the alpha wave state in your brain. The alpha state is when you feel relaxed yet alert as to what is going on around you. In other words, you are creating a calm state of mind so that you can focus effectively. Be sure to read this chapter all the way through before attempting any of these exercises.

1 Find a warm, safe, comfortable place, where you won't be disturbed.

2 Sit upright in a chair. Avoid lying down because we are conditioned to sleep when we do so. Allow the chair to support your body and sink into it comfortably.

3 Place your feet flat on the floor, with your hands resting on your thighs and allow your eyes to gently close. It is quite normal for thoughts to be drifting through your mind. Avoid fighting them.

4 Allow any external noises to drift in and out of your mind, whether it is traffic, people in the distance, aircraft, or a ticking clock. The secret here is to blend these external noises into this process of calm. For instance, you may internally suggest to yourself that as each car passes you 'melt' into a deeper sense of calm.

5 Slowly start to work down the muscles of your body – I emphasise the word SLOWLY. The mind needs time. Mentally take each group of muscles and imagine them becoming calm, floppy, at rest. Begin with the muscles of the face, including the cheeks, lips and jaw. Gradually move your attention to the shoulders, arms and fingers. Slowly move to the chest, stomach and back. Continue through to the thighs, calves and feet.

6 Once you have calmed your body but are mentally alert, count down from ten to one. Tell yourself that with each number, you will drift a little more deeply into a state of calm. Count a number on every other out breath.

7 Once you have completed the countdown, allow yourself to drift even deeper into a calm state. You have now engaged the alpha brainwave state successfully.

Practise this regularly until you can achieve a calm state easily. This is the state you should create within yourself before you use any of the following techniques. A simple way to do this and one which can help you to pick up the techniques quickly is to record yourself reading out points one to seven so that you are not distracted by reading them from the lines here.

Now, here are the techniques that will help you become the gorgeous, slim person you know you are. Feel free to use a combination of them; use the ones that work for you. But make damn sure you do at least one of them every day. Remember, only fat failures don't bother. All the techniques involve you closing your eyes and should be undertaken only when it is safe to do so. Before opening them again, always mentally count back up from one to ten. Tell yourself that you will open your eyes at seven and at the count of ten will be fully awake and that all normal sensations will be restored. Before fully awakening, affirm in your mind that you will wake up feeling refreshed, motivated, alert and ready for action.

> " If you suffer from epilepsy or clinical depression consult your GP before undertaking these powerful techniques. "

Technique 1

Begin by using the steps 1–7 above to access your alpha state. As you mentally count down from ten to one, imagine yourself becoming a little calmer yet more focused on each number. Then put the thought into your mind – and truly believe it – that you are a winner and that you are in control of your eating habits; that you are proud to leave food on your plate; that you are a no-nonsense Life Bitch success as you lose weight to gain a healthy shape. As you do this, sense the excitement it brings and in your mind hear the words 'being fat is something in the past'. You may even suggest to yourself that you are happy to be repulsed by being overweight and that weight control in your mind is a lifestyle change that you are immensely proud of. After ten minutes of affirming this to yourself, bring yourself back by counting up from one to ten.

Technique 2

Once you are in the alpha state, dissociate from your mind the part of you that thinks you are a failure when it comes to losing weight. Do this by breathing out the excuses and the victim thoughts and breathe in thoughts of achievement. In your mind, see, hear and feel the words FAT LAZY LOSING SLOB drifting away on each out breath. Then breathe in SLIM TRIM CONTROLLED WINNER. Let these words soak into your mind deeply. Do this ritual 20 times, finishing on a positive in breath.

Technique 3

This is the Life Bitch DIP formula. All three parts should be practised in the alpha brainwave state, but need to be learnt separately for some time before you put them together. Work through them as described below:

Define your vision

Drift into the alpha state and picture yourself in your mind as slim, relaxed, confident and comfortable with your image. See this success in a freeze-frame and take a mental note of the way it makes you feel. See it as reality now. Notice how proud it makes you feel. See what you see, feel what you feel and, if there are sounds, hear what you hear. As this is a portrait of success, you should turn up the brightness of the picture, intensify the wonderful feelings and by all means pump up the volume.

Spend around five minutes with your defined vision. When ready, count yourself up from one to ten in the normal way. Carry out the process for seven consecutive days.

> In my work with athletes, I get them to picture having gold medals hung around their necks before a competition has even started. They are first out of the blocks and over the finish line because they know they will win.

Identify the parts

Note down every action and behaviour undertaken that will help you achieve that ultimate vision of your ideal weight and body shape, and include all your positive verbal and non-verbal communication.

This could be something as simple as clearing the larder of biscuits, buying new outfits a size or two smaller, taking longer walks and constantly reminding yourself that you are a Life Bitch winner. In effect, these are all the consistent activities you will do to achieve your defined vision.

Having identified the actions that will help you achieve your defined vision, for the next two weeks, in the alpha state, see, feel and hear these 'parts'. Let these defined parts bury themselves deeper and deeper into your mind. In other words, let them become habits.

Play your success movie

Now bring together your vision with the parts that will make it happen and play them as a movie in your mind. Practise playing this movie for one week. Then use the movie when you are in situations that challenge your willpower, such as being out with the kids and everyone is having ice creams, or it's Friday night, when you usually have a curry (not anymore you don't).

The DIP technique will replace thoughts of temptation and craving with the real goals and outcomes you want: losing weight and being your ideal weight.

You will have conditioned yourself at the unconscious level to be in control, calm and focused, so that losing weight becomes a pleasure, not a chore.

Technique 4

I developed this five-minutes-per-day workout over a number of years and it is really suited to people who feel they need more motivation. It takes up very little time and delivers quickly. So there's no room in the Life Bitch programme for any fatties who say there's not enough time to work with their mind at a deeper level!

Relax and drift into your unconscious mind by closing your eyes and counting down from ten to one. Imagine going into the part of your mind that is the 'motivation room'. Drift into it and notice the sounds and feelings of powerful motivation. You are hearing shouts of 'Come on, you are a winner,' 'You are moving to lean arse and away from lardarse successfully.' Hear the roars of a crowd cheering you on. Let the motivation flow throughout your body. Imagine a sensation of win, win, win.

Finally, count yourself back up from ten to one. Increase the volume of your inner voice as you count up.

If you choose this technique, do it for five minutes every day, whether that be in the morning, on the way to work, in your lunch break or in the evening before bed.

Technique 5

Drift into a state of calm and imagine yourself walking down the street noticing lazy, fat people bingeing on food and feeling repulsed by them. Let that feeling of absolute disgust be your motivation. It makes you feel sick. Imagine the fat strangling their bodies and the emotional laziness these people have accepted into their lives. It is only fair to remember that not all fat people are fat because they are greedy – some have medical conditions – but the majority are fat because they are lazy and won't get off their big backsides to do something about it. You're not one of them anymore.

Technique 6

Drift into the alpha brainwave state and imagine a filthy tablecloth with a load of junk food on it. Notice the grease and stains on the cloth and feel repulsion as you look at mould and maggots on the fatty foods. Turn up these feelings of repulsion and the brightness of the scene. If there are sounds, turn up the volume. After a couple of minutes allow your mind to go blank. Then, in your mind, reset the table with a clean tablecloth and imagine white plates with healthy food on them; perhaps a serving of fresh vegetables with some lean chicken breast. Notice the colours and the feelings of freshness as they enter your mind. You could imagine the sound of your favourite music accompanying the scene. Allow this scene to enter your mind, deeper and deeper, and let it become your reality.

This technique and the one before will help programme your mind to control your eating habits, so you create the desire to eat small portions of healthy food. They will motivate your mind to be a slim, trim success, rather than be like the thousands who choose to remain fat slobs and continue down a lacklustre road to ill health.

Technique 7

This is one of the most straightforward of techniques. Affirmations are a way of working within your mind to change the negative pictures we have of ourselves to positive ones. Affirmations are simply positive self-talk, and affirmations linked with visualisation will support your quest for the body beautiful by improving your:

✓ eating habits

✓ approach to exercise

✓ personal projection as you shed the weight

The words you say to yourself produces pictures, which in turn will affect your actions and behaviours. Be sure to use affirmations both in and out of the alpha state. Remember to state them in the present tense and always make them positive:

✓ I love the feeling of my body as the fat dissolves

✓ I really enjoy the taste of healthier foods and the feeling that they are zapping my waistline

✓ I feel brilliant as I stride up the stairs to my office

✓ I deserve to strut my stuff and enjoy the confidence of success

✓ I look people straight in the eye and they can see the ray of light shining from me

✓ I am one hell of a successful Life Bitch slimmer

Technique 8

Using what is known as a timeline approach is a great way to absorb your new look deep into the unconscious part of your mind without the need to go into the alpha state. I particularly like this technique because it incorporates a bit of drama and gets you moving.

Find a space where you can visualise the journey of melting the fat. Mark a space on the floor that represents 'now' and stand there. With a real focus, walk from the 'now' space to a point on the floor that for you represents the successful you, looking fantastic and slim and feeling like the dog's bollocks. Stand tall on this space and turn around to look back at the 'now' space. Stay there for a moment, absorbing what it is like to have achieved this outcome. Feel what you feel, see what you see and hear what you hear. And now walk further forward to a space that represents the future, when you have achieved the body beautiful, and turn around. Take a look back to 'now' once again and visualise all the things that you did to achieve your outcome. Mentally talk to yourself, using past-tense language, such as, 'I stuck to my Life Bitch healthy menus, did some exercise each day and affirmed that I was totally in control of my eating habits.'

Using this technique, your mind will grasp that you are already successful. It will automatically programme itself to help take you along your timeline.

The good news is that by carrying out these techniques, the natural, practical actions you need to take to establish healthy eating and a healthy lifestyle will be automatically triggered because your mind will be motivated to carry them out. They are effective and simple: eating healthy food installs the habit in the mind and means you become strongly motivated to buy them.

These mind techniques will be the bedrock of your motivation. If you find yourself saying, 'I don't think it's working,' then get off your backside and try harder. You are dealing with the Life Bitch here, not someone who says, 'Never mind, it will happen one day, somehow.'

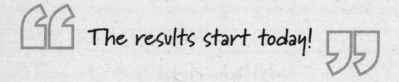

The results start today!

Trying harder means you need to focus on the mind techniques more. That's exactly what winners do. They practise until they reach perfection. Imagine a high jumper who decided to give up after they couldn't reach a certain height. The successful ones don't give up. They picture themselves clearing a height they haven't cleared before. They maintain the image of getting over the bar in their unconscious minds and keep practising until they achieve it.

Forget any silly excuses that may be going through your mind, such as, 'I won't have time because of the kids' or 'It's going to be difficult because I work long hours.' My response to this is, 'Loser!' I quickly get bored with all this hollow talk that today we work long hours and it's hard to maintain a work/life balance when you have children. What utter crap! Our ancestors would just laugh out loud at this attitude. They used to work just as hard, if not harder, than you do today and large families were more common. In the 'PC' world we live in today, the excuses are allowed to spiral out of control.

> So get rid of that fat-brained attitude right now!

> ## Real life
>
> Samantha had grown up in a family where meal times were a free for all, a bit like a pride of lions eating as much as possible, as quickly as possible before any rivals steal the food. As an adult, she felt it was important to pile her plate high and eat until she felt uncomfortably full. The result was that she was four stone above her ideal weight and deeply unhappy with the lack of self-control she had when it came to food.
>
> Working with Samantha over a period of weeks, I helped her reprogramme her unconscious mind using the positive disassociation [Technique 2] and DIP [Technique 3] programmes outlined above, so that she still enjoyed regular meals, but in much smaller portions.

Of course, these powerful mind-programming techniques will need to be done in partnership with practical actions. Let's consider these practical steps.

❗ The chances are you will regularly go to the supermarket. I want you to take great joy in skipping by the frozen chips and cream cakes you used to feel that you wanted. People in the supermarket may look at you a bit strangely because you've got a big grin on your face and a skip in your step, but just remember you are being a Life Bitch and so you don't give a damn what they think

- Use common sense when cooking your fresh food. Ditch the deep-fat fryer and use a low-fat spraying oil in the frying pan if you are frying food. Bake potatoes or cut homemade chips with the skins on and bake them in only a little oil

- When you are eating your plate of food remember that you can leave some. Give yourself a pat on the back each time you do this. It will condition your mind and body to start accepting smaller portions

- If you get a craving for a bag of pork scratchings or a frozen pizza loaded with meat and cheese, switch on the red stop sign and picture the disgusting lard that you would be putting into your mouth and adding on to your body

Real life

I worked with Jonathan for some time and he was a challenging subject to help move forward; not only was he fat, but he had a stammer. Both were symptoms of low self-confidence and so my job was to make Jonathan believe in himself and his abilities and programme his mind to disassociate negativity about himself when it came to overeating.

Life Bitch

Here's what I did with Jonathan:

I asked him to go into a relaxed state and in his mind picture a fenced-off area with a closed gate around him. I then asked him to use the power of his mind to open the gate and push through any thoughts and impulses that stopped him from controlling his eating and weight. In his mind, Jonathan saw these unhelpful and negative thoughts and impulses as red words which were pushed out as he breathed out. The words were things like 'curry', 'hungry', 'biscuits', 'snack time', and as he made a mental picture of these and physically pushed them out of his subconscious Jonathan felt the weight being lifted. As he breathed in, Jonathan was asked to think about words and phrases that defined his new confidence and control, such as 'ideal body image', 'slimmer' and 'proud to be in control'.

I sent Jonathan home and for five days he followed this reprogramming routine. Each day he spent five minutes in his alpha state doing this exercise. Soon he found that he had started to believe in his own brilliance and know that he could control his urge to overeat.

To strengthen his new self-belief and to help control his urge to overeat on impulse, I taught him another, quite tough, technique. I asked him to think about something pretty unpleasant while having snack impulses. The key was to get a gross image in his mind when the compulsion to snack came into his mind. What worked for him was imagining vomit over the food he was looking at or thinking about and then replacing those images with those of healthy foods. Jonathan lost over a stone in five weeks.

the
BITCH *list*

○ Practise the self-hypnosis techniques in this chapter to exercise your mind – it is your most powerful organ.

F**k the food

7

Picture the scene. You are walking down the high street; you pass some lovely clothes shops, book shops and a florist. At very regular intervals you notice the greasy kebab shop, the fish and chip shop, the additive-rich Chinese takeaway and, to top it all, the cholesterol-rich burger joint. You need to start noticing the healthier alternatives that most high streets offer when it comes to quick bites for lunch etc. Lots of places now offer salads and low-calorie sandwiches, juices and smoothies to give you the pep you need.

All the junk food outlets are a big temptation for the fatties who haven't yet taken responsibility for their weight problems and instead treat themselves to fish and chips with a kebab on the side. The odd visit to burger bars and open-all-hours fish and chip shops is cool with me, but frequenting them several times a week is not.

We are forever tempted with fatty foods and processed mush on the high street, TV commercials, billboard advertisements and internet pop-ups. It is for that reason that I am going to give you Life Bitch practical tips to avoid being tempted by this crap.

The dodgy server

Remember: people who work in fast-food outlets tend to be low-paid and not highly motivated. Their bosses are driven by profit and many have been caught out in the past cutting corners, especially when it comes to public health and hygiene.

So, next time you go to a burger bar, please note that the service assistant may have just returned from having a pee. And be aware that many public toilets fail to provide hot water and soap, never mind hand-drying facilities that actually work.

I remember my own horrible experience of visiting a burger joint in Malta. At the counter, I noticed the fingernails of my smiley server. Under his nails I could see grime, bogeys and other unmentionables.

I think I have made my point.

Diabetes outrage

The processed and fast food that is so easily available is devastating to our health if eaten to excess. The obesity that it causes can commonly lead to potentially life-threatening Type 2 diabetes.

In fact, if you are obese you are more than twice as likely to develop the condition than someone who has a normal body weight. The reason for this is that being fat puts added pressure on the body's ability to properly control blood sugar using its natural insulin and therefore it is much more likely that you will develop diabetes. The complications of the condition if it is not treated and managed properly are worrying, including blindness and problems with the feet and heart. And, most frightening of all, it is likely to cut eight years from your life expectancy, according to research by the University of Surrey.

As your Life Bitch, I think I need to point out to you that high levels of fat and sugar in processed and junk food will more than likely give you a very good chance of developing this worrying condition. Don't go there – follow the Life Bitch plan.

Look at the queue

Next time you are in town, take a look at the crew in the queue at the chip shop. I would estimate that over half shouldn't be there because they are obese. Imagine those that shouldn't be there completely naked. What a ghastly sight! Watch them wobble to the car, struggle to get in and take a good look at their huge arses.

People become obsessed with takeaways and junk food and crave the bucketloads of salt and fat that they contain. I remember once when I was in a chip shop – yes, I do on the odd occasion go into them – there was a really fat guy who came in and, with great pride, ordered a large portion of chips and two steak and kidney pies to go with them. I thought, 'What a greedy-guts,' but I was even more shocked when the girl behind the counter said they had run out of his favourite pastry-topped savouries. The look of worry on the guy's face was ridiculous. He had to cancel the order and turned to his wife and said, 'Don't worry, we'll go to the chip shop at Spark Hill instead.' Get real, people!

Be repulsed by the thought of feeding on fat. If you are ever tempted to join the fast-food queue too often, just grab hold of some of your excess flesh and let this motivate you to go buy a smoothie instead. You don't want to become a figure of fun, like the guy frantically making his way to the chippie in Spark Hill.

Think the stink

I want you to pay as much attention as possible to the smells of fatty fast foods. Let the disgust feed your mind. In fact, to create a real aversion to such fatty, smelly foods, you may want to imagine being sick on the food itself, as my client Jonathan did in the 'real life' example on page 92. I remember going for a walk with Andrew, another client, when we came into close contact with what I will call a 'processed food' factory. The stink was cheesier than cheese. Andrew suddenly stopped, went a strange colour and puked up all over the path. I guess it's not surprising that he never ate cheese again. Allow yourself to be angry with those that want to feed this trash to you. Then smile and affirm that you are in control and say two powerful words to these producers. 'No thanks.' From here, immediately allow your mind to wander on to some of the pleasant, fresh food scents you come across in life: mint, lemon zest, tomatoes, melon, fruit juice and homemade bread.

Shopping cheats

Sod the 'two for one' offers that bombard you as you walk down the food aisles. You may think you are doing the right thing by stocking up on an extra packet of frozen burgers for the family, but the price in terms of health is too dear. Isn't it nice of these food companies to help us to further clog up our arteries?

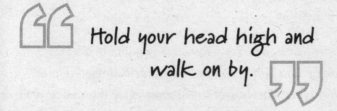

Hold your head high and walk on by.

Show them what you are made of by stocking up on what makes you a Life Bitch winner – fresh fruit, vegetables, lean meats, fish and wholegrain cereals will give you and your family a healthy future.

Take it away for good

You've become addicted to your Wednesday, Friday and Saturday night takeaway treats. Have you any idea about the empty calories, additives and dodgy hygiene practices that throw themselves up when you tuck into another takeaway meal? I used to wonder if leftovers from the night before had ended up in my takeaway and who may have sneezed over my so called 'treat'. When this struck me as a possibility, I threw out all the takeaway menus and decided this was a case of my own survival.

I want you to:

! Go through your kitchen drawers and look at your pin boards. Grab the takeaway menus, rip them up and throw them in the bin. You'll get rid of the temptation of having rubbish food delivered to your door when it should be delivered straight into the trash

! Walk tall past the takeaways that you come across regularly and if you decide to stop and smell the food cooking, imagine being overpowered by the stench until you vomit over the food you are thinking of buying. Start to associate the overused-cooking-oil smell with the smell of vomit and you will break the habit

! Keep a tin in your kitchen and every time you are tempted to buy a takeaway, put in the money you would have spent. Pretty soon it will mount up and you will be able to put it towards buying some of the fab new wardrobe that you will need when you've lost loads of weight following the Life Bitch programme

Journal time

I want you to review what you've learnt from this chapter on how to avoid the pitfalls of fast and processed food. Take out your Life Bitch journal and note down the feelings, fears and hopes that it has evoked. Write down the affirmations that you are going to practise to help resist the temptations that may have become embedded in your lifestyle.

Do this and it will give you another firm foundation to move forward on the Life Bitch journey to a slim, trim you.

the BITCH list

- Remember the dodgy server!
- Have a blood test to check you are not diabetic.
- Let the big buggers in the queue turn you off.
- Train yourself to be turned off by the unhealthy food you once loved.
- Forget the processed-food special offers.
- Get rid of your takeaway menus.

the BITCH list

- Record in your journal your thoughts and the actions you need to take to avoid processed foods.

Food and exercise: the right stuff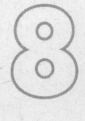

Now you've started to programme your unconscious mind to think healthy, to think slim, to believe in a new you – a you who is a winner – you need to ensure that your conscious mind knows the part it has to play. You've installed positive messages about achieving fitness and a slim, trim figure, but now what?

It's all about taking action. To help you, here is my three-week, get-yourself-started plan. But be warned: once you embark on this, you'll have to say goodbye to something that you've nurtured – all that fat you've so carelessly piled on. You'll have to take responsibility for who you are and be a winner. The good news is that now you have programmed your unconscious mind to support you in your quest to become slimmer, the conscious actions you must take to be healthy will be a lot easier.

Life Bitch

Life fuel, not fat fuel

Your first task is to plan your daily menus for the next three weeks. Why three weeks? Well, it takes about 21 days for a new habit to be formed.

> " The habit you are going to form is one that will ensure you are slim, trim and not ready for the mark-down bin. "

Start believing that preparing your own meals only takes a little thought and a decent recipe book, even if you are not an experienced cook. I know you will enjoy cooking your own food; it will help relieve stress and will give you a sense of achievement. More than anything else, cooking your own meals shows that you are in control.

As I said before, I'm not going to give you a diet to follow – what you eat is your choice; how much you eat is your choice – but make sure that what you put into your mouth and the amount you put into it supports what you believe in your mind: that you eat healthily, you eat to be slim, you eat to be the you that you want to be, the real you.

Most of you will know the sorts of food that never satisfy your hunger and keep you fat – doughnuts, crisps, cakes, sweets, sugary drinks. I could go on and on, but you already know all the usual suspects. Many of you will also have read enough diet books to be experts in what not to eat and drink. You should already have a good idea which foods help you to maintain a fabulous figure, a bijou bum and solitary chin. But let me remind you of just some of the fabulous options available from which to plan your three-week menus. My list is based on plain common sense and hasn't been taken from any of the diets out there.

- **Vegetables:** broccoli, cabbage, carrots, kale, asparagus, mangetout, courgettes, aubergines, mushrooms, spinach, sprouts, squash, pumpkin, potatoes (baked or boiled), green beans, sweet potatoes, leeks, garlic, fennel, turnips, swede, shallots

- **Salads:** tomatoes, lettuce, celery, onion, beetroot (not pickled), bean sprouts, radish, peppers, cucumber

- **Fruit:** (always fresh rather than tinned) grapefruit (the Life Bitch says try to start a meal with grapefruit as it can help burn fat), apples, pears, plums, melons, oranges, grapes, blueberries, pineapple, bananas, strawberries, raspberries, mango, cherries, kiwi fruit, olives

Life Bitch

- **Meat:** lean chicken breast, canned tuna in brine, tuna steak, lean ham, turkey breast, turkey mince (can be used instead of beef mince and it's a lot less fatty), lean cuts of pork, fillet steak, fresh fish – especially white fish

- **Other proteins:** tofu, pulses, baked beans, cottage cheese, nuts (not roasted or salted)

- **Carbs:** High fibre cereals (avoid those with a high-sugar content – the Life Bitch recommends Weetabix or porridge oats), wholemeal bread, brown rice, wholemeal pasta

- **Misc:** low-fat spread, low-sugar jam, Marmite, low-fat yogurt, low-fat salad dressing, low-calorie dips, homemade soups, soy sauce, herbs and spices, instant gravy from a bouillon cube

- **Drinks:** water (the Life Bitch insists on a minimum of eight glasses a day), diet drinks (in moderation), fresh juice, skimmed milk, green tea, fruit tea, decaff tea and coffee

This list is clearly not exhaustive, but it gives you the general idea – and, let's face it, you do already know. You don't have to cut out anything altogether, though, and you shouldn't shy away from the occasional treat: a small takeaway (not an extra-large meal, or a 12-inch pizza, deep crust with extra topping!), a regular-sized chocolate bar, a cone of chips, a couple of glasses of wine – **but only every now and then**.

> Eating is a pleasure, but don't let the pleasure principle take over.

What to do on special occasions

If, during the three weeks, you attend any special occasions, such as birthdays or weddings, just use your common sense and be disciplined about how much you shovel on your plate at the buffet table. It's easy to spoil for yourself what should be a pleasant occasion by constantly being anxious about food, and it's equally easy to use the occasion as an excuse not to start your three-week plan or to sabotage it. Use plain common sense in selecting the types and quantity of food you eat. Portion control is your responsibility. The Life Bitch suggests a small portion would be a tea cup not a mug.

Dos and don'ts for special occasions

1 Remember that temptation will be put in your way and that you can pull out the red stop sign if you are about to lose control.

2 If you are about to fall by the wayside and eat something that you really shouldn't, use one of the powerful disassociation techniques discussed earlier, like imagining the vol-au-vent covered in vomit before it goes near your lips.

3 Have a treat – a glass of champagne, a small piece of cake.

4 Take pride in your self-control and smile at your achievement.

5 Get off your arse and have a dance if there's the opportunity, as it will burn off the celebration food you've enjoyed in moderation.

6 Don't say 'Screw the diet' before you get to the occasion. This is extreme weakness and I won't tolerate it.

7 Don't get smashed on any free booze as you'll then feel more inclined to tuck into large quantities of unhealthy food.

Never say diet

Remember: in my opinion you don't need a commercial diet plan, with recipe after recipe dictated for you that include ingredients that you've never heard of and that you can't find in your local supermarket. You don't need to be told what to eat; you already know. It's simple, so no excuses.

" If you have a medical condition, please consult your GP before starting the three-week plan. "

The three-week food plan

Okay, now I want you to plan your three weeks of fabulous, appetising menus. Remember: don't go into starvation mode. Make sure that you eat three meals a day – breakfast, lunch and dinner. It's just a question of thinking simply and thinking ahead. If you really don't have a clue where to start, take a look at the sample daily menus on pages 239–251. The secret is to plan your menus to sound tasty, exciting and more appealing than that bag of chips or piece of cake. You may be worried that you'll feel hungry during the day. When you're eating a healthy, well-balanced diet of three meals a day, hunger is mostly in the mind, but when I was losing my excess flab, if I was still genuinely hungry between meals, I snacked on fruit, vegetables or nuts.

Regardless of what menus You plan, the Life Bitch has some Ground Rules for You to follow:

! Grill, don't fry

! Drink a pint of water before eating

! Use a smaller plate than normal

! Snack on fruit

! Slow down as you eat: chew like you've never chewed before

! Leave some food on your plate and be proud of it

Here are some additional practical tips:

1 Buy one of your favourite types of melon and have a quarter or half of it for breakfast one morning, spruced up with some fresh ginger. The next day, use the remainder for your lunch to form the basis of a fresh fruit salad with some strawberries and pineapple

2 Roast a chicken and have some of it for your dinner with some really nice, crisp vegetables, such as French beans, broccoli and courgettes. Eat the leftovers the next day in a salad with a few olives and sun-dried tomatoes.

3 Take some fresh salmon fillets and coat them with a little salt, a drizzle of olive oil and some fresh basil. Pan-fry the fillets and have one for dinner and keep one in the fridge to flake into a green salad for your lunch the next day.

4 On Saturday morning, round up what remains of your weekly supply of fresh fruit and blend them together with a hint of honey and natural yogurt. You've got the perfect smoothie and a great way to start your weekend.

Exercise

A common-sense and controlled approach to food is only one weapon in the armoury you will use to fight fat. Exercise is another, so now let's get your body moving.

It may have been years since you have bothered to do any form of natural exercise. I don't mean going to the gym and becoming a Muscle Mary, I simply mean getting your body moving or, less politely, getting your arse off the sofa.

 Burn off that fat!

Life Bitch

It won't be just the crap food that you've shoved in your mouth that's made your pot belly blossom or your thunder thighs expand or your chin develop brothers and sisters; it'll be because you haven't got off your fat arse and done some exercise.

So what can you do to change this?

Feel the burn

I can hear you: 'Please, Life Bitch, no burn. I'm too unfit.'

I'm not talking about jogging for an hour and not being able to walk the next day. Oh no, you are going to start small and work up to the big burns.

Firstly, forget joining a gym. Many overweight people join with good intentions to attend regularly, but after the initial wave of enthusiasm fail to keep it up. And that's if they even start to go at all.

The Life Bitch prescription is as follows:

Stage 1

- Start walking, rather than taking the car, when you pop to the shops

- If you get the bus regularly, start getting off a stop or two early and walk the rest of the way home or to work or wherever you are heading

- Three mornings a week, get yourself out of bed early and go for a 45-minute walk before you start your working day. This may sound like a lot, but one or two of the days could be non-work days. If you feel that it is difficult to motivate yourself to walk for walking's sake, maybe your walk could have a focus, like going to pick up your newspaper, or taking the dog for a walk

- Five evenings a week, go for another 45-minute walk

- Take the stairs rather than the lift whenever possible

- Have a dance to your favourite music when you're cleaning

- Don't shop on the net. Go out shopping

Stage 2

- Consider going on bike rides. This is something that you can get the whole family to take part in

- Exercise aerobically for a minimum of 200 minutes a week, and avoid letting two consecutive days pass without taking such exercise. Use a couple of hefty cans from your larder as weights to get the arms and heart going. Try it before breakfast and just before dinner to burn up calories before you eat.

You see, there's nothing hard in any of this; the key is to

DO IT!

Real life

One of my clients, Gemma, has come full circle from being slender to a self-confessed fatty, and back to slender. She put on the bulk when she started to spend more time with her kids and got into home-cooking (and eating).

Gemma has taken control of her eating habits and has literally danced off the excess weight. She said, 'I really wanted to celebrate getting thinner,' and what a way she found through dance, something that gives her a brilliant aerobic workout and lets her exuberance and sense of fun shine through.

The dancing has been combined with thinking sensibly about menu choices, especially when she dines out. Gemma will check there's something delicious to eat, but be careful not to make it calorie heavy.

Another one of Gemma's practical hints I like is to simply make sure you don't go for long periods without eating and then make the fatal mistake of stuffing your face when food comes your way. She eats before going to a business reception, for example, knowing that she might go without any food for hours and then be offered plates of tempting, calorie-rich hors d'oeuvres.

One of her other little secrets is to break the weight loss down into achievable goals and rewards, so, for example, she buys herself some new clothes after losing 15 pounds, arranges a special getaway after another 15 pounds and so on.

Gemma's weight–loss journey has inspired me to put together some tips based on her sound advice.

1 Do cook with your kids, but focus on healthy eating.

2 If you are going out to a restaurant where you know there will be loads of calorie-rich dishes, have a little something healthy before you go. If you are a regular customer, pre-order something healthy before you get there, so you don't end up drooling over the menu.

3 Spend a few moments to think about a sport or hobby that you have always wanted to do and set aside some time to start doing it as soon as possible. This could be netball, salsa dancing, ice skating, flying a kite – just use your imagination.

the BITCH *list*

- Eat for the need, not the greed.
- Use your common sense to work out what foods you should and shouldn't be eating.
- Don't let special occasions ruin your good intentions.
- Forget about faddy diets!
- Plan some delicious, healthy menus.
- Haul your fat arse off the couch and start to be more active.

Booze busting

D on't skip this chapter if you don't drink because you can evangelise the Life Bitch approach to keeping alcohol in proportion to others. Let's face it, some people just don't know when enough is enough, and then they end up looking like a complete turkey and are full of regret the next day.

 If you feel you might have a problem with alcohol, seek professional advice now.

Booze hound or sensible snifter?

Gauging if you are drinking too much or drinking a sensible amount per week is tricky because it depends on factors such as your size and metabolic rate, but let's look to the Department of Health for some basic guidance. They say a sensible amount is no more than two to three units of alcohol per day for women and three to four per day for men (two units is equal to a 175ml glass of red or white wine or a pint of standard bitter).

I'm not going to preach to you as someone who's teetotal and despises alcohol in all its wicked forms – I like the odd glass of Pinot Grigio or champagne – but if you are a fatty and you drink, then you need to cut down your alcohol intake as part of your Life Bitch programme.

Take a look at the calories you can consume through booze alone. It's scary! A 175ml glass of white wine is 150 calories and a pint of cider is a whopping 250 calories; a few of these every day and you stand little chance of losing weight because you've drunk the calorie equivalent of scoffing a whole Indian takeaway with naan bread in a couple of drinks! The other scary point is that after a few drinks you will probably want that whole takeaway to yourself anyway because alcohol sharpens the appetite.

Binning the booze

My approach to getting you to cut down on your alcohol intake is simple:

- Firstly, make sure you don't drink every day of the week – have dry nights for four out of the seven

- Limit your booze intake to getting close to the daily recommendations if you are way above them at the moment, or to the daily recommendations themselves if you are not

- Don't try to be clever by saving up your weekly allowance for a blow-out on a Saturday night. You will harm your body and be the centre of everyone's fun, with people laughing at you rather than with you

- If you are going out with mates for a big night, make sure you drink plenty of water and switch to soft drinks after you've had your daily allowance. Feel proud of yourself that you don't need to match your friends drink-for-drink and ignore the drains who will say you are a 'lightweight'. That's exactly what you want to be

Are you binge drinking?

If you are binge drinking, and by this I mean going well beyond the daily alcohol guidelines for men and women on a regular basis, then take a cold, hard look at yourself when you are sober.

To overcome the binge-drinking habit, I want you to do the following:

Step 1: I want you to form a mental picture of yourself when you are at the height of your lack of self-control – perhaps you're being sick, having to pee in the street or stuffing a greasy kebab down your throat. Whatever it is that you end up doing because you've had too much alcohol and it has dulled your senses and made you lose all self-control, see yourself doing it and be disgusted. I want you to be truly repulsed by these thoughts and images of yourself, because you damn well should be.

Step 2: Before you next go out socially, count down from ten to one and then picture yourself smiling and joking at the bar with a glass of fruit juice in your hand. Come out of your self-hypnosis session by counting from one to ten and saying to yourself, 'I'm relaxed,' 'I'm happy,' 'I'm looking forward to meeting my friends.' By using this technique, you will feel relaxed and you will not need alcohol to bring about a perceived state of calm in your mind.

Let me be direct with you. Who is really going to be impressed with a beer-swilling, wine-guzzling, tummy-bouncing fatty at the bar? What's more, if you are out on the pull beware, because if you get lucky and spend the night with someone you are more than likely going to be snoring, farting and, if you are a man, suffering from penis malfunction. Folk do talk, so beware of having a reputation as the one that can never get it up!

Combine the self-relaxation technique above with some self-discipline and, whether you are out drinking or at home, have one or two alcoholic drinks but no more! Keep in control and then switch to soft drinks and water to keep you on the straight and narrow.

Alcohol has its own rewards

Yes, it's widely acknowledged that alcohol in moderation, especially red wine, has some health benefits, but let's keep it in perspective. Like the processed food that has become a problem for many of you, alcohol is relatively cheap and easily available. You can get it delivered with your food shopping and there are now around-the-clock pub hours, but do not use these as excuses to drink too much.

> Spend a little more than usual on a good vintage wine or a nice bottle of bubbly and share it with friends. That way You won't drink to excess and because of the good quality, You won't want to. Think of this as a reward for being a great Life Bitch and sticking to Your target.

Real life

I'm not going to pick out an individual for a real-life look at the impact of alcohol on weight loss and weight gain; I'm going bigger, much bigger in fact, and looking at an entire country. It's nice to bitch about a group of people who tend to do a lot of bitching about others themselves — in this case, the French.

I read not so long ago in the Daily Mail about a study which 'exploded' the myth that all French women are thin. And it's not only that they are eating the wrong foods, a lot of them are drinking like fish, or should I say poissons. The study found that just under 20 million of the 63 million population were too fat and the growth trend was worst among women. Imagine my surprise when the article said that one in 30 French women are drinking so much that they would be classed as alcoholics.

Even in France, where home-prepared food was once as sacred as the ritual of eating around a table, the worst aspects of modern culture have taken hold — too much processed food, cheap alcohol and more McDonald's than anywhere else except for America.

This was shocking news for me, but given the trend for binge eating and drinking in the UK, perhaps it shouldn't have been.

Go back and look at the Fat in the Frame chapter where I talk about role models. Your lack of control when it comes to drinking alcohol sends terrible messages to children and young people. I find this deeply worrying. It's up to you, as adults, to do something about it.

> " To the booze hounds:
> alcohol has its place, but don't
> let the drink become your
> master and you its lap dog. "

the BITCH list

- Know and respect your healthy daily limit when it comes to alcohol.
- If you are a binge drinker, use the self-hypnosis techniques in this chapter to end this disgusting behaviour.
- Give yourself a small allowance of the best alcohol you can afford as a treat for reaching milestones on the Life Bitch programme.
- Use your common sense when it comes to alcohol and be a positive role model to others, especially young people.

Fat child of mine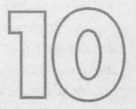

If you have children, or close contact with kids through family, friends or work then this chapter is of particular significance to you.

We've all read about the obesity time bomb, the issue that is now one of our biggest collective health concerns, but have you stopped to think that you can guide your children so that they don't fall into the obesity trap? If you haven't, then wake up and smell the coffee – start to think right now that it is your responsibility and nobody else's.

When I see fat parents sitting stuffing their faces with burgers and chips in front of their children, I cringe with disgust and sadness. These parents are simply giving the green light to their kids to go through life choosing the easy, unhealthy options when it comes to food.

If you are one of those failing parents, shape up and give your jaws a rest for a change. It is your job to be a positive role model, one that demonstrates that weight control isn't hard, isn't a chore and isn't something that should take the pleasure out of life.

Come to your senses because the truth is that if your kids don't control their weight they may be bullied at school, face discrimination when they go for job interviews, suffer ill-health and ultimately die early. You made the decision to have kids, so it is your job to look after them. Face up to your responsibilities right here, right now.

This doesn't just apply to parents; it applies to grandparents, uncles, aunts and anyone else who is in a position to be a positive role model to a child. I don't have children, but I sure do see it as my duty to shine as a healthy role model to my nieces and nephews. I give them healthy food such as fruit, vegetables, wholemeal bread and so on, but I also treat them to an ice cream if it's a special occasion. They learn from me and their parents to appreciate food as fuel for the body and enjoy the taste of good, fresh food.

Becoming a role model

I want to give you a set of Life Bitch tips that will allow you to set a brilliant example to your own children and all those who look up to you. Make these part of your Life Bitch mission; help your kids to become slim and, most of all, stay slim.

1 Debunk the junk. Throw away the crisps, biscuits and junk food that are in your cupboards. Let your kids watch you do this and take the time to explain why the empty calories end up becoming a chain that drags you down. Have fun as you do it. Ask the kids to smash up the trash food and throw it hard into the bin. Tell them you are planning to change the way you eat by using your common sense. As you do this, show them excitement and joy that comes from eating common-sense foods. Let them know that you don't need to watch programmes telling you what to eat to be slim, as you already know what you have to do. Yes, it's back to damn well using your common sense.

2 When you have dumped the rubbish, take the time to sit down with the kids and play the Life Bitch menu game. Explain that you want them to use a common-sense approach to eating healthy foods and invent a Life Bitch menu using these principles. Show them the Life Bitch menu examples on pages 239–51 and get them to have a go at drawing up their own menus. Praise them and take them shopping to buy the ingredients they need to prepare their menus with your help. Tell your children the old adage that 'food tastes much better when you've cooked it yourself'. Put their menus on show in the kitchen and take some pictures of the dishes they enjoyed preparing, to act as inspiration as they progress.

3 Never, ever let your kids see you shovel heaps of junk food down your throat. I was in the high street recently and saw a young woman pushing a child in a pushchair while scoffing a huge burger. Do you honestly think it was only I who felt disgust? No, of course not. Here was a woman wearing clothes that didn't do her justice – the rolls of flesh dribbled over her waistline and her bottom looked as though it could be used as a flotation device. There are plenty of bad examples of adults gorging on junk food everywhere you go, but enough is enough. You are a Life Bitch role model who has to reject this. See that red stop sign in your mind if you are ever tempted to stuff garbage into your mouth, especially in front of the kids.

4 Don't be a losing, lazy lump and order your food online to be delivered to your door. Not only does it show your children how bone idle you are, but it removes the beneficial physical activity associated with shopping and takes the kids even further away from the reality of where food comes from. This is a big no no for the Life Bitch. When you do need to go food shopping, get your kids to help you put together a healthy list of food that you will all enjoy and if possible take them with you to pick the items and carry them home. Perhaps use a points chart, scoring each item they suggest a mark out of ten for healthiness. If they do really well, reward them by agreeing to take them to the cinema or a trip to Alton Towers in the school holidays. It's not difficult, is it?

5 Kids should know their way around in the kitchen. Have them help you to prepare healthy meals and get their hands on fresh fruit and vegetables. Have fun with them and they will understand you are a Life Bitch champion. Avoid shouting at the kids if they make the odd mistake in the kitchen. You might even pick up some creative ideas from them. I remember my niece once teaching me how a little shredded carrot in a fruit cocktail adds a crunchy, fruity feel. She didn't get that from a book either.

6 You might have seen those disgusting images of mums passing their kids burgers, chips and pies through a school fence in South Yorkshire. This is an unforgivably bad example to kids all over the country. All parents have got to encourage their children to eat balanced, healthy meals, not a pile of crap in a polystyrene box. Make sure you support your school in providing your kids with healthy school dinners. Thanks to Jamie Oliver, local authorities, schools and parents have acted to improve the nutritional value and quality of school meals, and what we don't need are parents sabotaging this great effort.

7 Get into the habit of showing your kids that it's okay to eat ice cream and chocolate occasionally, but not too regularly. Let them know that popcorn and ice cream is okay on a trip to the cinema, but that then it's back to following the Life Bitch's principles. I never advocate denying kids the occasional treat, but I do advocate making the time to serve your kids healthy meals. I really don't want to hear excuses such as, 'It's hard to find the time,' 'They are picky eaters' or 'I want to give them the food that makes them happy.' They are the future, so take the time to put fresh, healthy food on their plates and teach them that real food is fun. Just get off your arse and do it!

8 Something that many parents have lost sight of is the importance of active play. Children need at least one hour per day of decent exercise, and don't rely on their school doing this for you. It's all too easy to allow your kids to sit in front of the TV or play video games in their rooms for hours on end. You have got to set an example and get them outside and active, having fun and learning that daily physical activity is essential. Go for a bike ride or have a game of football, swingball, badminton or Frisbee. Teach them how to play golf, take them out for a long walk with the dog or set up a game of hide and seek in the park. There is no end to the fun activities you can do with your children. Not only will you all be burning calories, but you will also bond as a family unit. Most children will be reasonably able in at least one sport; if your child is good at something, nurture their talent and reward it. If, for example, they are passionate about tennis, pay for coaching, or if they are football crazy, get them involved with a local youth team.

I hope you now understand just how important your role is in helping your children develop good eating and exercise habits. It's vital that you make the effort. Use the 'real life' examples below as inspirations.

Real life: Julia and William

Julia, 37, is a single parent with one son, William, aged 12.

Julia wanted to be slim and so did her son, who was around two stone overweight. It really hit home when on a holiday William took off his shirt and was embarrassed about his shape in front of other kids. Julia knew then that something had to be done. Together they planned healthy menus and went shopping for ingredients, and she made it all fun for William by introducing a points-for-health system.

Even though she worked full time, Julia made sure that she spent time with her son in the evenings, doing practical tasks that contribute to healthy eating and a balanced lifestyle. She would set up a rewards scheme for William if he replaced the junk food he loved with healthier alternatives. Together they planned and set the rewards from buying him a basketball to redecorating his room together, as well as taking him for walks at weekends to his favourite park. They planned a six-month strategy to condition their minds for health, fitness and slimmer figures.

Within three months, they had both become trimmer and slimmer; it was success all round. Further down the road, both are still firmly in control. William is doing well at school and Julia reports a massive improvement in his confidence.

The Archer family

Martin, 48, and Sonia, 43, were both clinically obese. Martin had a heart attack and survived, and this was the wake-up call they both needed. They jointly came to the realisation that their three children Oliver, 13, Claire, 9, and Tom, 6, were becoming lethargic and fat.

Their first step was a conscious decision to increase physical activity by going camping and walking in the countryside as a family. This step up in family-focused physical activity was married to an agreement to immediately cut by 50 per cent the amount of takeaway meals eaten by the family.

As an additional boost to the upsurge in physical activity, the family agreed to start shopping together. They found they had fun buying food for the healthy meals they had planned, and were burning calories by getting out and about.

They launched 'Operation Fat to Fit', putting up pictures in their kitchen of healthy food and of families having fun and being active together. The three-month programme of introducing common-sense food and exercise choices, planning varied and tasty family meals and sustainable weight loss has paid off: a total of 89lbs of family fat was successfully shed in the three-month kick-start campaign to lose weight.

An agreed incentive is helping their motivation to stay slim. If after 12 months their weight is still at healthy levels, the family will go to Euro Disney for a week.

Sally, Dave and Samara

Sally and Dave are friends of mine. A few years ago they adopted Samara, 15.

Samara had grown up in a country with a completely different culture and set of life values. She was a normal, healthy weight when she was adopted, but within a couple of years of starting school in the UK, she had become obese, largely through spending her dinner money on chips, crisps and chocolate. The situation got so bad that she was sneaking chocolate into the house and helping herself to goodies from the larder.

Realising that Samara had started to eat far too much fat and sugary foods, her mum and dad decided to help her get back in control with some sensible eating. They talked to their daughter about why she was eating so much junk food and the answer was simple: it was something that was completely new to her, her friends were eating it and she liked the taste. Mum and Dad explained that she couldn't eat junk day in, day out and that they would all work on a healthy-eating programme.

First, they arranged for Samara to start eating school meals and agreed that only a small proportion of her pocket money could be spent on sweets each week. Next, they encouraged her passion for horses by arranging for her to do some part-time work at a local livery yard.

Sally and Dave rewarded Samara for sticking to their agreed healthy-eating plan with pieces of riding gear, from a hat to a new pair of boots.

Samara found that she had got back to a healthy body weight within four months and that she had a natural gift for working with horses.

the BITCH *list*

- Encourage your kids to help you throw out the junk food in your fridge and cupboards.
- Plan some delicious, nutritious Life Bitch menus with your children.
- Take the kids to the supermarket and make a game out of shopping for healthy, common-sense foods.
- Have fun in kitchen with your children.
- Don't deny your kids an occasional treat.
- Get active with your children.

From fatwalk to catwalk

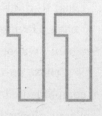

The Life Bitch is conscious that you have put in a huge amount of effort to slim your body down. On your journey, you will have had dreams of the clothes that you really want to be seen in. Let's talk fatwalk to catwalk.

Now the time is right to get your image just as you want it to be. It's time to glam up. You can now wear the clothes that make you look gorgeous, move like a sex machine and ooze so much panache that it's difficult to imagine that you were ever fat.

Praise be that the days have gone when you wobbled down the road, completely out of puff. It's time you conjured up the image of you walking down the catwalk.

Life Bitch

You've earned it, so I want to pass on to you some top Life Bitch advice about how to get your outward appearance right.

Several years ago, when I managed to leave behind my fat suit, I had to think long and hard about making the most of my new image. Having lost 36lbs, I wanted to look handsome and sexy again, I wanted to make the best of what I had.

I chose the clothes that suited my body shape, found colours that complimented my skin tone and flattered my features and selected classic pieces that would form the basis of my wardrobe. I was also aware that I had to have the right clothing for the right situation, so that I was always projecting an image that was bang on.

Moving from fatwalk to catwalk made me feel simply fabulous. Gone were the days when people blew raspberries behind my back and so-called friends told me that I had nothing to worry about regarding my obesity. I increased my confidence, flirted more and achieved things in my life that I had only dreamt of before. My career took off and I found my soul mate. The point I am making here is that your appearance contributes massively to how successful you are in moving your life forward in other key areas outside weight loss.

> I dumped my fat and I look great. Now it's your turn.

Take stock of three core areas: the dress check, the appearance check and your persona check.

The dress check

Now the time is here for you to look in the shops for the outfits you never dared to wear before. Whether you like it or not, the clothes you wear create an overall image that others will judge you by in just a matter of seconds. In other words, the way you dress will determine 'brand you'. Brand you is everything from your personality to your appearance, but it is the latter that we are concentrating on here.

But before we go any further, have a clearout right now of clothes that are associated with you being fat. Put them in a bin bag or three and take them to the local charity shop.

When shopping, box clever and try to go for the best quality you can afford above quantity. Treat yourself to clothes made from good fabrics that won't easily crease and buy simple, classic, well-cut garments. Perhaps buy yourself two or three quality outfits that can be mixed and matched with other clothes, but that form the basis of a classy, chic wardrobe. I want your clothes to make you look like you are an exclusive designer label in your own right, rather than a bargain-basement sale item.

It may have been a while since you took a real interest in the way you dressed, so here are some Life Bitch dress-check tips:

Life Bitch

▌ Check what colours suit you. Ask a shop assistant for their candid opinion, or consult a friend. If you really want to splash out, hire an image consultant

▌ Think really hard about your image and the way you want to look in different situations – at work, when out socialising, on special occasions. For example, if you are going for a job interview wear a smart suit that's cut to accentuate your best bits and choose some simple accessories that will make you subtly stand out from the crowd. For the girls, this could be one or two pieces of jewellery, such as a necklace that draws attention to a lovely neck or a nice belt that shows off your slimmer waist. For the guys, consider a double-cuff shirt with some swish cufflinks (nothing naff like boxing gloves or sports cars!) and a tie that draws out and complements details in the shirt and suit. If you have any doubts ask your nearest and dearest or a friend for an opinion on your choices

▌ Make sure your shoes are polished and that they match your outfit

▌ Get inspiration on what's hot from the fashion pages of good style bibles like *Red*, *Grazia*, or *GQ* and *Esquire* for you guys

! Keep a note in your Life Bitch journal about what clothes have made you feel really great and which outfits have picked up the most unsolicited compliments. This will do you the power of good

The appearance check

Once you've sorted out your wardrobe, it's time to take a look at your personal appearance, so you can make the most of the fab clothes you are now wearing. By appearance I mean everything from your scent to your hairstyle.

The good news is that when you were fat you probably had to apply masses of deodorant to combat your body odour, but now that you are much fitter and slimmer you will be far less whiffy and can think about perfumes and colognes. It is also highly likely that you didn't pay much attention to your hair, make-up or nails – and, guys, this applies to you as well.

Let's go through the list of Life Bitch appearance tips.

! Your hairstyle should be a priority. Go to a salon for a free consultation. For years you may have let the hair fall like rats' tails or stuck to a safe Purdy cut or the same old colour. Well, as a Life Bitch, it's time to get it right. Go to the best quality stylist you can afford. Make sure you give your stylist an impression of the way you really want to look. Look through magazines to find pictures of styles you think will suit you and take them with you when you go to the salon

! As well as the hair on your head, make sure you control your facial and body hair. Keep your nasal hair and those long, bushy eyebrows trimmed, clipped and plucked. There's nothing more off-putting than meeting someone for the first time and they've got facial hair sprouting out of places it shouldn't be

! Now for those nails. Keep them clean, tidy and manicured. There's nothing worse than shaking someone's hand and seeing a load of accumulated grime under the nails; it makes you wonder what on earth they've been doing

! When it comes to scents and colognes, go for something that matches your spirit and personality, and, whatever you do, don't splash it all over, so that people are bowled over by the overpowering fragrance. If you are buying a new scent, ask a friend for their opinion. Once you know which scent best suits you, stick to it

! We all hate being near people with bad breath, so take care of your oral hygiene. Clean your teeth regularly, especially after meals, and avoid eating food with strong flavours if you are going to get up close and personal with people you want to impress. Keep a breath-freshener about

Get Off Your Arse and Lose Weight

your person. Now that you are smelling fabulous take
yourself off to a store that offers make-up demonstrations

! Think carefully about your skin and make-up. Take
yourself off to a store that offers free make-up
demonstrations and let a professional advise you on what
really works for you and your image. Like everything
else, it's all about common sense and often less is more

! Fellas, it's not uncommon to see guys with make-up on
these days, but if that's not your cup of tea, at least make
sure your skin is in good shape. Use quality moisturisers
and shaving balms to calm down razor burn and take
care of those pimples and blemishes

Your persona check

This is where you are going to see a vast improvement, Life
Bitches. Now that you are losing the chubs, your body glides, your
smile radiates and your physical animation excites. Your persona
is going to be magnetic. You are going to give men a hard on,
women the come on and yourself the good old 'bring it on'.

Develop some Life Bitch success habits when it comes to the way
you move, talk and pose. Don't be surprised to see fat people on the
periphery looking at you with envy. They want what you've got.

Life Bitch

! You probably didn't think about it when you were a chubby, but you need to be aware that the way you carry yourself speaks volumes about you. Take a moment to become aware of your posture. Walk tall now that you are not curved over by all the excess fat

! Go out of your way to observe the way slim people stand, sit and walk and try to imitate them. Use the power of your imagination – pretend you are walking down the catwalk or the red carpet at a celebrity bash

! Make yourself more animated by using gestures. The movement of your arms will add clout to your persona and the impact you have on others. This will be easy now that you have moved away from being a resident of chubby land. Your gestures will make others interested in you and help you communicate more fully. For example, in a bar talking to a stranger you may say, 'I think it is important for people to take personal responsibility and just go for it.' On the word 'responsibility', point towards yourself. On the words 'go for it', open out your arms, palms up, and shake them a little. These small gesticulations will add flavour, colour and excitement to your persona

! Your facial expressions are going to be much more interesting now that your blubbery cheeks have shrunk and your eyes can be seen more clearly. Remember –

and this isn't really such a cliché – the eyes are the doorway to your soul. Making eye contact with others is crucial. It will tell them that you are confident and interested in them. Combine great eye contact with facial expressions that will light up the room with your newfound confidence. Think proud thoughts about yourself and smile and flirt with your eyes. Eye contact will not only make you look confident and sincere, it will create an intimacy that you may never have experienced before

! Your voice can at last project confidence. It's time to make the most of your vocal equipment, be it at the office, in the pub or in the bedroom. Watch you don't go over the top, though, as this can be irritating. Train your voice to sound confident by practising this simple exercise. Imagine a situation you need your voice to project, such as a blind date, a job interview or asking your boss for a raise. Both sitting and standing, try out different volumes, paces and inflections to develop emphasis and distinction. It pays to exercise your vocal muscles as much as your body muscles in order to communicate effectively

Real Life

Bret was a 45-year-old divorcé. He blamed pigging out and becoming podgy on his failed relationship. In all he piled on three stone and reported a complete lack of self-worth. He emailed me to ask for support and I informed him that there would be no crying over spilt milk (full-fat, of course) and that he would be directed to make immediate changes without digging his heels and throwing tantrums.

Wanting to be more confident with people after losing his fattiness, he concentrated on developing his outward appearance. He worked on putting together a wardrobe that suited his character and ambitions. Part of this involved writing down the most common situations that he found himself in, from going to work to going out on a blind date. Together we looked at picking out the clothes that would make him stand out as a smart, switched-on guy. The results were amazing; he went from humdrum to stunning Brum with a few careful choices of jackets, shirts and jeans.

We then moved on to working on his body language and making sure he used eye contact to his advantage. Looking people in the eyes had been something this man hadn't done well for years. Bret practised and practised until his eye contact became what I call a conditioned response. I practised gestures with him and even asked him to chat me up! He did very well. Bret started to attract more attention to himself and went on to get a promotion at work and buy a new apartment where he could entertain his ladies.

Amie

Amie was a 32-year-old dumpling who ate herself into such a state that she was unable to fit in an aeroplane seat. She took control and sought advice from the Life Bitch. A combination of the mind-control techniques you have learnt and getting off her backside to exercise allowed her to shed an amazing six stone. Naturally, she then wanted a man in her life. To achieve this, we worked hard on developing strong body language by using gestures and got her into the habit of visualising herself engaging confidently with others. Decreasing weight and an increasing persona led her into the arms of a man five years her junior, and a bit of a hunk, I have to say.

the BITCH list

- It's time to glam up, so start making an effort.
- Show off the new you by buying some flattering, good-quality outfits.
- Take pride in your appearance. Get a new haircut, sort out that unsightly facial hair and pamper yourself with a manicure and some new make-up.
- Think about how you present yourself to others. Stand tall and proud, project your voice, make eye contact and use body language to put your personality across.

Seasons to be bitchy

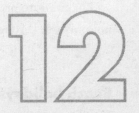

If you are wondering how you are going to cope with the weight- loss pressures and temptations of the beach holiday, the spring weddings, the summer balls and the Christmas party season, then I have some advice for you. I want you to use your common sense and dig into the Life Bitch techniques we have developed together.

 No bullshit excuses.

These situations are often a real challenge for wannabe slimmers and, boy, do they get overly dramatic about them! Yes, we do normally celebrate with food and booze at these seasonal events, but your Life Bitch power is going to be so strong that these situations are going to be a breeze for you.

I'm going to provide you with tips and tactics so that you will not only get through these occasions, you will also enjoy them.

Beach holidays

Yes, if you are going on a beach holiday, you will feel the pressure. You will desperately want to bare some flesh, but feel that you can't let the folds feature. But get over it because you are with the Life Bitch, and next time you go on holiday you will be slim and gorgeous.

Preparing for the holiday that you deserve should include packing a number of your Life Bitch tools. Take the following items with you:

- The sexy beach bikini you are going to slim into

- Your list of Life Bitch affirmations

- Life bitch menus. If you are taking a self-catering holiday, follow them as closely as possible. If you're not cooking for yourself, look at them to remind you of the kind of food you should be ordering in restaurants

- Your Life Bitch journal

- A gross picture of you at your heaviest weight
- This book – your weight-loss lifebelt

As soon as you arrive at the resort, place your Life Bitch affirmations in prominent places around your villa or hotel room, so that you can easily read them. If anyone in your party thinks you have gone a bit strange, just tell them that you most certainly have – it will take the wind out their sails every time. Place your hideous fridge picture somewhere in the room where you are going to see it constantly. Perhaps place it on the bathroom mirror or in a frame on your bedside table.

You are going to enjoy your holiday so much more knowing that you are in control and are continuing to shed weight.

Hang up that bikini in pride of place in your bedroom so that you see it when you get up in the morning and when you go to bed. Enjoy the self-belief that the next time that you come to your favourite holiday resort you will be able to wear it. Let this bikini inspire you every day while you are on holiday, knowing that you are losing the 'fat duck' label and really going for that transformation into the beautiful 'slim swan'.

It's not nice to see all those jelly bellies tanning up in the summer sun, but I want you to have a peep. There is nothing wrong with looking at the beached whales as you walk along the beach or by the pool. Let it remind you of what you will become if you end up caving in to the pressure to try real Madeira cake or the range of local cheeses.

Life Bitch

It is hugely tempting to consistently overeat on an all-inclusive holiday, where you can eat and drink as much as you can possibly get inside you until you fall over. Keep centred in your mind the thought that you are a true Life Bitch as you choose a small plate and refuse to pile it as high as Mount Vesuvius. In many cases, the alcohol will be 'free'. Yes, it's free from a monetary point of view, but the real cost is the damage to your health and weight. If you feel tempted to join others and drink until you are sloshed, take a look at your Life Bitch journal and read about your commitment to stick to the daily alcohol guidelines.

If it was up to me, these ridiculous eat-to-excess holidays would be completely banned. What a bad example they set our youngsters, and no wonder the number of obese people is starting to outweigh those who have a healthy body weight. All they do is encourage people to get as fat as possible. But not you, my Life Bitch star, because you know better.

As you enter the dining room, step away from the holiday treats – ice cream, baklava, chocolate pudding, cream with your strawberries and so on. Be strong and choose the lower-fat and lower-sugar options, like sorbet and naturally sweet strawberries without cream. Ask yourself, 'Is this platter going to make me fatter?' If it is, then it is simple – say 'no'. Picture that slinky, sexy bikini.

At night, dance until you sweat in the humid heat. Drink plenty of water, and remember: no binge drinking, please. I want you to visualise yourself next year, strutting your stuff on the dance floor in a sexy little number that will turn heads. For you guys, imagine losing the *cerveza* gut and spare-tyre hips, so you can hold your head high on the dance floor.

The wedding slimmers

Got that hat? Outfit at the ready? Is the weather looking good? Attending someone's wedding is great, but the amount you eat and drink can become a stone around your neck if you let it. Here are a few tips to avoid pigging out, toasting the happy couple too often and saying 'yes' to those desperate to buy you a drink.

At the reception, take the arrival drink and move on through. Gently sip rather than throwing it down your neck. If another is offered say, 'No, thanks.'

It is now time for the sit-down meal. Engage in conversation with those at your table and don't be afraid to let out your charm. You are becoming more charming by the day as a Life Bitch role model, so enjoy it. Eat slowly and make sure you leave some of the food on your plate. Sip your wine and mentally remind yourself that you are firmly in control. Have a glass of water at hand and take sips of this at regular intervals. As you look over at 18-stone Uncle George scoffing his third buttered roll as though tomorrow won't arrive, let this reaffirm your success.

Getting through the speeches can be so dull, if we are honest. Do you really want to know the details of how they met, what it will be like with a new son- or daughter-in-law and how beautiful

17-stone Sarah looks as the bridesmaid? As the toasts come and go, be in the habit of raising your glass without sipping a drop. Watch the other sad buggers swallowing the lot and requesting another glass.

As the early evening disco begins and Uncle Stan starts to dance like a runny blancmange, watch with a sense of fun. As others join him, get on the floor and strut your stuff. As you heat up feel the calories burning away.

It's 9 p.m. and the lights come on. It's buffet time, and the queue gets longer and longer as a row of salivating porkos just can't wait to get a plate full of pie, chips, quiche and bread. Pop to the bar at this stage for some water and when the queue has eventually shrunk go up and get a nice plate of salad, a few sandwiches and some fruit salad to follow. If there isn't any fruit salad, take just a small portion of dessert. Avoid denying yourself; just let your newfound control allow you to say, 'I'm satisfied.'

Bounce with joy at the summer ball

Charity summer balls are more popular than ever and the chances are that you will be asked to attend one. You'll face the welcome drink as soon as you walk in, smell the wonderful dinner and feel as though you are about to fall off the Life Bitch wagon. Well, you're not going to because I won't let you.

Well before you attend the ball, get extra motivation by asking family and friends to sponsor you to fit into your dream ball outfit. This extra support and the chance to donate to the ball's nominated charity will really get you going.

You are wearing your dream outfit and you have a real bounce in your step, not from the fat you used to carry, but from the joy of knowing you look fantastic. As you take your welcome drink, enjoy the slimmer you and the attention you are getting from people who have not seen you in recent months. Talk to them, while taking small sips of your drink, and savour the compliments you are getting, not the fizz you are drinking.

> Be the belle of this ball; the Life Bitch is really proud of you.

Christmas parties

Working on preparing your mind can help loads with combating the festive parties and their negative implications for people losing weight. You need the ability to avoid the booze, Christmas cake, sausage rolls, pork pies and chocolate truffles.

In November, begin affirming to yourself, while in the alpha state, that you are in control, and visualise yourself looking and sounding totally in control. Bring in contrasting thoughts about the losers who say, 'I'm starting my diet in the New Year.' I bet they say this every Christmas and have been overweight for years. You already know that the Life Bitch bans the word 'diet', so just smile internally when you hear them say it and remember that you are losing weight in a long-term, sustainable way.

When you attend these parties, take your hideous picture with you. Trot to the loo occasionally and take a look at it. Let it remind you what's going to happen to your body if you give in to a moment of weakness. There's no way you are going back to the time when you struggled to find clothes you wanted to wear that would fit you.

If there is someone at the party who catches your eye, make sure you go and talk to them. As you engage in conversation (with naughty thoughts in your mind), keep mentally reminding yourself that in all likelihood they are not attracted by a sumo-type figure.

When it comes to the food, design your plate of food to look like you enjoy food, but not too much in comparison to the skyscrapers that the others seem to have built and are demolishing all around you.

If possible, plan to drive home, so that you can't drink alcohol. In fact, volunteer to be a nominated driver. There'll be no peer pressure because the pissheads will know you are doing them a favour.

If you *are* going to have a few drinks, dig into your resolve and make sure you limit yourself to a couple of glasses of wine or single measures of spirits with low-calorie mixers.

Enjoy the party and be reassured that you are brilliant for doing things the Life Bitch way. If you have been following my programme for some time, then don't be surprised if a stranger requests a kiss under the mistletoe!

Now you can let invites to social events bring a big smile to your face and reinforce your motivation to be a Life Bitch slimming success.

the BITCH list

- Stay strong when faced with temptation and pity the whales that shovel it in.
- Remind yourself of the slob you may become by looking at your worst picture at times of weakness.
- Eat slowly, sip gently and remember that you are in control.
- Enjoy!

Life bitch: the three-month audit

If you are a true Life Bitch, then you will have stuck with all the techniques explained in this book. If you did, then well done you, and I hope you've rewarded yourself along the way.

If you have fallen off the Life Bitch wagon, stuffed your fat face again and feel a bit of a failure, then I want you to know you are right – you are a true failure. But there is a way back on to the Life Bitch weight-loss wagon. Just read on.

I am going to give you six Life Bitch actions to help you get back on track.

> **Not only will you get back on that wagon, you will be its driver.**

Life Bitch

Carry out the following Life Bitch actions and stick to them tighter than those leggings that make you look like a whale. This is the last-chance saloon for those who have fallen down, and there is no margin for failure. You have got to give this your all or just walk away now.

Before you go through the steps please get the tears out of the way. Yes, you failed and that was down to you, so don't bother blaming anyone else. Just get on with it right now, please.

The actions

Action 1

Email the Life Bitch at info@lifebitch.com and let him know that you are firmly in the driving seat and that there is no going back. This will show that you have some commitment to the action plan. Explain to me what life is going to be like when you are a sexy princess or stud once again. Give me details on why you have not kept up with the Life Bitch weight-loss programme and affirm what you want to achieve and how you are going to get there. Believe in yourself that you can do this. It is the first step you need to take to catch up with the wagon, so let's keep rolling in the right direction.

Action 2

With immediate effect, carry out the following mental exercises:

! For three days, dissociate the pathetic mental states you have not yet got rid of. I am calling them pathetic because they are; they have constantly held you back. And, be honest, you agree with me, don't you? All the excuses and claptrap about being weak and craving certain foods are to be ditched. Imagine them flying into a bottomless pit, never to be seen or heard from again.

! For three days after you have dissociated these warbling excuses, place the success outcome in your mind by seeing it, feeling it and hearing it. Enjoy this process because it is shaping a new, confident, slimmer you. Picture your success, the glamorous image you will have and the fun, parties and sex you will enjoy as you hit your ideal weight.

! From then on, affirm to yourself powerful messages that your situation has changed for the better and that when it comes to weight loss you will never allow yourself to be a brain-dead, losing, whining victim again. Instead, you will be a Life Bitch king or queen, who holds their head up proudly and looks people in the eye with confidence.

Action 3

Go out for a walk down the high street and look at the fat people. Look at the family of fatties getting into their car. Look at their spare tyres, droopy arses, floppy bingo wings and multiple chins. See the car sag as it struggles to take the strain. It's sad and revolting – this is not for you anymore.

Have a look also at the snail-pace that fat people walk at and how this irritates other pedestrians. They do this because they aren't able to shift their fat arses at a reasonable pace anymore. Feel sorry for these people and really install in your mind how you will be like that if this time you don't succeed on the Life Bitch journey.

Finally, stop by one of your former fast-food haunts or cafés and see those fatties stuffing down bacon butties, chips and fried chicken. See the grease they lick from their lips and imagine it sticking to their hips. Enough is enough – you are dropping the fat suit right now. Remember that your excess fat is just a suit that you can choose to take off; underneath is the true you that is dying to see the light of day.

Action 4

Make a timetable of the walks you are going to take in the next month and put it on the wall. Plan these walks for early in the morning, to show that you can get out of bed. The walks should get longer in distance and become more intense. At the end of the month, remember to try to take yourself to the top of a hill, to signify the height of your achievement and your new outlook on the world.

Make sure you get the revolting picture of yourself back on the fridge if you have taken it off. And now find more of these fatty pictures and put one in the bathroom, one in the bedroom, one in the car and one by the front door, so that you see it whenever you leave the house.

Action 5

Plan your menus as usual, but this time take your time with them and produce a portfolio, something you are really proud of. Plan them for four weeks this time, and think about planning your success dinner party and the special but healthy meal that you will share with your friends.

This is your own à la carte Life Bitch menu-planner. If you think one of your menu ideas should be shared with the Life Bitch army, send it to the Life Bitch himself at info@lifebitch.com.

Do not, whatever you do, blame other factors for your lack of weight control! It is all down to you. You always looked to blame others for the reasons why you overate, but in truth you knew it was down to your own self-control. Nobody else pushed the food down your throat.

You are either going to stay in control as the driver of your Life Bitch weight-loss wagon and drive it with a full, clean licence, or you are going to rack up penalty points until you are banned altogether. Believe me when I say that I have no time for you if you collect points on the licence and will welcome you being banned from driving your Life Bitch wagon if you are a weak-willed, moaning victim.

On the other hand, if you are a successful, slimming winner, I welcome you as part of my army. Completing this journey means you are a role model and a friend of the Life Bitch. Well done!

the BITCH list

- Get back on that wagon right now and stop whinging.
- Email the Life Bitch and let him know that you are committed to the programme.
- Observe the pathetic fatties in the high street – you don't want to be like them anymore.
- Timetable your daily walks and make sure you damn well stick to it this time!
- Put some real effort into planning your Life Bitch menus.
- Remember that it's all down to you, so just get on with it.

Living proof

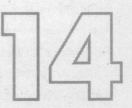

Does the Life Bitch way work? You bet it does, and I'll prove it by citing three of my success stories.

Puddings to lean machines the Life Bitch way

In December 2006, I agreed to let the BBC film the Life Bitch in action. I was so convinced that my approach worked that I was willing to test it out in a prime-time evening slot. My first task was to find willing volunteers, so I advertised for participants. I needed to find a few guinea pigs I felt I could work with and who had the strength to take it the Life Bitch way – hard. Having advertised, I then auditioned would-be Life Bitchers, ultimately selecting four people. The challenge I set myself and my participants was to get them to lose an average of at least three pounds per week over the three weeks of the programme.

I needed to be assured that my Life Bitches in the making were willing to provide at least 50 per cent of the motivation needed to complete the programme; I'd provide the rest. I was looking for people who had mental stability and who obviously needed a change in lifestyle, people who wanted to move from being weeble wobbles to pert pinups. The applicants had to convince me, in no uncertain terms, that they deserved my time.

My labfats

The people I selected had all tried lots of different diets, which of course hadn't worked. This time would be different. My methods would work, and in the three weeks they were with me, I would set them on the road to a new lifestyle – one of energy, personal control and success.

These people had no medical condition or deep psychological trauma that they could use as an excuse for being fat; they'd simply become lazy and sedentary and, in a way, had given up. That was until they met the Life Bitch.

Let me introduce you to my laboratory fats:

⚠ **Andrew** was 47 years old and weighed 21 stone 1lb. Simply through being lazy, he was not shedding an ounce. He looked like a bubble – it was a bubble I was going to burst. Andrew explained to me that he wanted to be 12 stone 7 pounds. He claimed he'd tried Slimming World, WeightWatchers and Rosemary Conley – all good programmes – but, for some reason, he remained fat.

I agreed to provide him with three weeks of no-nonsense Life Bitch motivation to kick-start him – and, believe me, the emphasis was on the kick.

Kate was 25 years old and, simply put, she was enormous. At just under 19 stone, she had eight stone to lose and, to be quite honest, without the Life Bitch style of motivation, in my opinion, she hadn't a hope. She had as much chance of losing weight as a chocolate éclair had of remaining in her fridge for more than a day. To make things worse, she explained that she hadn't eaten a single vegetable for ten years.

Well, the Life Bitch was going to take care of that. It's amazing what being blunt with people can do. I was going to make her realise that she could eat vegetables and enjoy them:

Sandra was 56 years old, a bubbly extrovert and a highly emotional character. She explained that she had tried Weight-Watchers, Atkins, Slimmer's World and Rosemary Conley, but she still had four stone to shift. In other words, through her own lack of effort and focused motivation, she had failed.

Sandra was about to receive the biggest caning she had ever known from the Life Bitch. I was to realise from working with Sandra just how much people can enjoy a bit of caning!

Life Bitch

The three-week programme, covered by the BBC, would include menu planning, the application of clinical hypnosis, time with the Life Bitch personal trainer to get them moving again and a direct, no-bullshit approach. We also had to come up with a lifestyle plan that they would continue on after the conclusion of the three-week programme.

Let's have a look at what they did and didn't do.

Andrew DID

- have several takeaway meals a week
- have a long, lazy lie-in every weekend
- have a stomach so big it was doubtful that he could see, let alone tie, his shoelaces
- stuff chocolate, crisps and sweets into his mouth when watching TV (which he did a lot of)
- try commercial diets, and failed every time
- keep moaning about being too fat (and probably got on everyone's nerves doing it)
- reward his sedentary lifestyle with more food — it's a good job his local store was well stocked
- have a family history of heart disease

Andrew DIDN'T

👍 go for gentle walks to work off his flab

👍 eat using his common sense

👍 get strong and take responsibility

👍 see the many people around him who took the mickey
out of him for being so fat

👍 bounce back, even though others could bounce off him

At one point in my initial interview with him, he came close to tears; he had a 15-year-old daughter, he told me, and it was his ambition to one day walk his daughter down the aisle on her wedding day. At the size he was, he was afraid that he'd embarrass her or maybe not even be around when that day came. He wanted to be slim; he wanted to be fit.

He agreed that he would take on my non-politically-correct style and shut up moaning, get working and do this for himself.

I discovered that Andrew was a keen singer with an amateur dramatics group. That was good news – to be so actively involved in something in his spare time showed that he could muster self-discipline and apply himself to a task when he wanted to. Very soon, I decided, he would be singing 'Take My Breadth Away' instead of 'You Can Leave Your Fat On' and 'New Pork, New Pork'.

Life Bitch

Kate DID

- 👎 shovel in several chocolate bars and bags of crisps a day
- 👎 try the odd diet for a few days, but would very soon give them up
- 👎 recall when she wasn't as fat, but unfortunately the memory was fading into the dim and distant past
- 👎 recognise herself as a fat and lazy slob
- 👎 catch sight of herself in the mirror and instantly try to cover up, reaching for what would have to have been a very big towel
- 👎 try to squeeze into that special dress, but often found it would show every bump and bulge. Eventually, when she stepped into it it didn't even make it past her thighs

Kate DIDN'T

- 👍 do any exercise at all. Occasionally she would promise herself she would do some tomorrow, which of course never came
- 👍 eat vegetables at all and ate only tiny amounts of fruit
- 👍 take enough responsibility to just get on with it and lose some flab
- 👍 know what it was like to feel successful and in control of her weight

Kate arrived at the audition for my Life Bitch programme looking a little shy and timid, but behind her eyes I could see a real determination to succeed.

She explained to me that when she was thinner she used to skydive. Looking at her size, I thought that if she did this now, then heaven help the person she might land on. She told me that she loved it and really wanted to skydive again, for charity. It didn't take me long to realise that this young woman, once she'd heard my messages and been on the receiving end of the Life Bitch motivation programme, would soon be whittling away the fat and become a skydiving diva once again.

Sandra DID

- own over a dozen exercise videos, but looking at her, I knew she never used them
- try umpteen different commercial diets, none of which got her to her desired weight
- in the past get initially excited about losing weight, but soon lost that burst of enthusiasm, never lost weight of any significance and gave up
- have a routine where she ate bagels when she got in from work, followed by a full dinner and then a binge-out while watching the soaps — a fantastic recipe for piling it on
- want to look sexy in tight jeans and brown boots, but was too lazy to do what was necessary to achieve this

Sandra DIDN'T

👍 bother thinking about eating common-sense foods that would help her melt away the fat so that she could get sexy again

👍 have an ounce of motivation for the long haul

👍 live in the real world. She thought weight loss would one day happen, but failed to accept that it wouldn't happen through a miracle and that she would have to make it happen for herself

Sandra saw an advert for my Life Bitch programme in the local paper. She finally took positive action and turned up to my audition. She walked into the audition room, sat down and then screamed at me, 'I want to do this! Accept me on this programme!' Sandra's emotions were clearly running high. I made her work hard at the audition, asking what *she* would do to make it work for her. I demanded that she take my messages on board and told her there would be no excuses allowed once she had signed up. The strength of her feelings convinced me she was right for the Life Bitch way. It was time to make Sandra sexy again, and I was going to do it.

Life Bitch winning formulae

From the very outset, I told the participants that if they were going to whine and be serial complainers, I would have no time for them. My time would only be given if they deserved it. Now was the time for consistent effort on their part – a bit here and there would not be sufficient. I also told them that I expected to see smiles on their faces, as the time they spent with me would not be doom and gloom; it would be three weeks of celebration.

So, as you read this book, put a smile on your kisser. You have a good reason to, because at last, you've found your path with the Life Bitch way.

My next lesson was to get my role models to feel repulsed by fat, and especially their own fat. I wanted them to see their fat for what it was – ugly and unhealthy. There was no room in my programme for them to pretend that their excess weight was a result of past emotional turmoil. In fact, I pointed out to them that many slim folk are just as likely to have faced deep personal problems.

I made them find a picture of themselves looking fat, one which repulsed them when they looked at it, and then stick it on their fridge.

A central theme for the three-week programme was to install success habits into their minds by using self-hypnosis. I ensured that none of the participants was epileptic or suffering from clinical depression, and so they were all able to undertake these exercises.

Over a three-week period, they practised the techniques described on pages 77–88. The aim was to encourage these people to get in touch with their positive inner voices. Over the years Andrew, Sandra and Kate had done little to change their failure states, so it was no wonder that they were losing the battle to melt the fat; in other words the loser talk they were giving themselves had become unconscious; I was going to change all that. Motivation was going to be drilled into their heads, come hell or high water.

I was going to make motivation an automatic response for them. They were going to learn new success habits and make these a normal part of their everyday lives. What they thought, felt and did would automatically make them thinner.

I expected these new success habits to be visible in their homes; this included positive statements plastered on the walls and food in their fridges and cupboards that would drive them to slimness. I demanded a weekly timetable of exercise. They were told I would not accept weak excuses for not doing one hour's exercise a day, which in this case was walking briskly, to burn the fat. The exercise also included picking up litter in a local park – a bit of bending and stretching is something that's good for all of us. The positive statements they pinned up on their walls were things such as:

I am a Life Bitch winner.

I am in control of my eating habits.

I am melting the fat from these flabby buttocks.

I am going to enjoy flirting as the new me.

All three bought pedometers to make sure they were walking enough. All able-bodied people should do 10,000 steps a day, but these guys were told to increase this by at least 20 per cent.

You too should go out and buy a pedometer, but if you are unsure about your ability to exercise or you have high blood pressure, take advice from your doctor first.

The role models were then directed to think about something that they could go out and buy which would act as an inspirational tool for them. Perhaps something expensive, something that would make them look and feel great when they slipped into it. They each also went out and bought an item of clothing two sizes smaller than their current measurement and were told to hang this up where it would be constantly seen.

The participants were told to throw out any clutter which, in my opinion, could hold them back, clutter such as exercise videos, diet books and any other so-called slimming aids that in the past had made absolutely no difference to them other than creating a sense of failure and dismay. On a visit to Sandra, I encouraged her to rip up a 'diet card' from a time when she was a member of a slimmers' club, where everyone used to sit round talking about how 'good' they had been – or in many cases, not. As she ripped it up, she became a real Life Bitch role model, saying that this stupid weight loss group had been full of whinging people who needed to get a life and just do it. It was at that point that I knew Sandra was getting rid of her old dead-end habits.

Over the three weeks, the theme of 'no excuses' continued. I carried out spot-check visits to my role models and if the actions I had ordered them to take weren't happening, I made it clear that their blubber would remain.

> Take note because blubber will be the most outstanding feature of your body if you don't act.

They were all told to look out for people who were being irresponsible. For example, if they witnessed a fellow lardy going into the chip shop, they were to think, 'Get your fat, binge-eating, lazy arse out of there, you stupid sod.' If you find this comment offensive, then good! Perhaps you will be shaken into action for a change. I've always said that restaurant doors should be a certain width, so that if any able-bodied person can't fit through them, they won't be allowed in.

All the role models were instructed not to step on the scales for the first two weeks of the programme. If you are one of those people that continually weighs themselves: GET A LIFE! Jumping on the scales every day reeks of desperation. And anyway, weighing yourself once every two weeks will excite you much more when you see the weight you've lost.

Next, the Life Bitch role models were told to inspire three other people around them to take the Life Bitch approach. Sandra, in particular, rose to this challenge, telling her family to start taking responsibility, to get out and walk and to get motivated or stay fat. This is what you should be doing. To inspire others means you are reinforcing your own worth and your success habits.

After two weeks, I allowed them to step onto the scales. I was there to witness the results. Emotions ran high. Sandra screamed, 'Yes! Yes! Yes!' and punched the air as she realised she had dropped ten pounds in two weeks. Next up was Andrew, who welled up when he saw that, at last, his body had shrunk by eight pounds. Finally, it was Kate's turn. Her confidence had begun to build up and she looked radiant when the reading showed that she had shed ten pounds. Amazing results.

During the final week, all of my participants continued their regimes and I asked them to work even harder. I demanded that they all lose one stone in weight by the end of week three. Thereafter, it would be down to them to continue their significant weight loss and weight-controlled lifestyles. The established norm for long-term weight loss is one to two pounds per week, but the Life Bitch way naturally sheds the weight more quickly in this intensive three week kick-start. All confirmed that they were still working with their unconscious minds, programming in adverse reactions to fat and planting success habits.

I constantly reminded them, via emails and home visits, that people who moan and do nothing are obese in attitude as well as body, and that those who are action-machines are the ones who get sexy, trendy, healthy and feel alive again.

The results

After sticking to my programme for three weeks my role models were happy to find that:

- their stomachs were travelling from fat to flat
- their confidence was climbing high
- their success habits were well and truly in place

Let's see how each of the participants did overall:

Andrew

Andrew's final result was excellent. At the end of the three weeks he weighed in at 19 stone 6 pounds, a massive shift from his 21 stone 1 pound – a loss of 23 pounds or well over a stone. In a single week Andrew dropped 15 pounds which is radical, but not surprising given that he was so overweight. Fantastic! Naturally, he was delighted with this loss of lard, this blasting of the bloat.

Andrew said he found the programme easy to follow. In fact, he enjoyed the challenge. My way to health wasn't too prescriptive and, using the power of his mind, he was able to approach the whole experience positively. He was driven to make common-sense choices about what he ate. He found that through the use of self-hypnosis, he didn't feel hungry. He never felt he hadn't eaten enough. He found he was able to go from breakfast to lunch without wanting to snack; the food he ate was keeping him satisfied. In particular, he found the technique of associating unhealthy, greasy food with letting his daughter down. In fact, he found that the greasy smell of this food actually made him heave. He was able to associate food-fat with own fat. This was good news; his unconscious mind was updating itself – new files were being installed, old ones deleted.

Andrew found that the hardest part of his new lifestyle occurred in the first week, when, because of many years of inactivity, he found the walking hard. He experienced pain in his legs and got blisters on his feet, but it wasn't long before this got better.

I asked Andrew if it was simply the changes he'd made in his food consumption and his new exercise regime that had helped produce his dramatic weight loss or whether other factors had been important. He replied that other key factors had helped his motivation and determination. These he discovered thanks to my support. With my motivation methods, the key message had penetrated his sluggish mind: 'Get off your arse and work it off!' He had found my regular text messages to him urging him on to success particularly helpful. Andrew had begun to welcome the challenges he faced, was keen to continue and was already looking to the next hurdle.

This was not difficult to anticipate. Over Andrew's three successful weeks, he had had my support, my nagging and my no-nonsense straight-talking to urge him on and keep him on the right path. Now he had to go it alone. Had the three-week programme been enough to change his habits long term? I asked him exactly what he would be doing to ensure continued weight loss. Successful though he had been, he was still a long way off his desired weight. Andrew said that he was determined to work hard and carry on with the instructions and advice I had given him. He felt that he now had the support of those closest to him and that this would help.

Andrew's colleagues had noticed and commented on the positive changes they had witnessed, and this had been a great extra motivator for Andrew. He also told me that others had been interested in the programme he had followed – he had inspired them. And it wasn't just that he looked slimmer and healthier; there were additional benefits from following my programme. His psoriasis had begun to clear up and he felt more energetic and less stressed. He said it was as if he was constantly detoxing his body. And if these changes weren't enough, he also felt more confident. Not only did he feel in control of what he put down his gullet, he also felt more in control at work: he found he worked more quickly and efficiently and his faith in his own judgement had improved. Andrew now trusted his own decisions and no longer dithered or constantly questioned himself.

Andrew had introduced a total change in his lifestyle. He felt so positive that he was inspired to inspire others; his belief in the benefits of the programme was absolute.

In my last session with Andrew, I gave him the following advice:

! He should continue with his self-hypnosis. I stressed that he needed to keep this up or risk going backwards

! He should keep the repulsive picture of himself on his fridge door and his positive affirmations on the walls

! He should picture two scenes. In the first scene he was to imagine his daughter getting married. He wasn't present – his unhealthy weight and lifestyle had brought on his premature death. Although this was in many ways a happy day for his girl, she also felt deep sadness at his absence. I told him to use his imagination to create the scene, to really see it, hear it and feel it, as if it was for real. He was then to pause and let his mind go blank. Next, he was to picture a second scene – a more positive picture. He was to see his daughter's wedding day again, but this time Andrew would be there – fit and healthy – and would be part of the celebrations. For this scene, he was to turn up the brightness and feel a heightened sense of it

Kate

Starting out at 19 stone, Kate finished the three weeks at 17 stone 8 pounds. It was amazing to see a bubbly, very pretty woman emerging from her podgy prison. It was clear that Kate would be turning heads soon. In fact, she had already noticed admiring glances coming her way and her confidence was cooking. She knew she was moving from deep-frying to high-flying.

I asked Kate what the main thing was that had made this programme work for her. Without hesitation, she said it was the mind techniques and, in particular, using the mind to focus on what is good and bad food. She also said that she had not found the programme difficult to stick to and that the whole process had rapidly got easier, mainly because it made her feel good; this new lifestyle she was treating her body to felt very natural to her.

Hunger wasn't a problem for Kate, and after meals she felt full. There were some temptations along the way, however. As she worked in a nursery, there was often cake or chocolate available to celebrate birthdays. How did Kate cope? She used her mind, as I had advised her to. She would imagine something like baked beans or vomit poured all over the tempting, sugary offerings and as a result had absolutely no desire to eat them – well, would you?

Kate clearly found the three-week programme more effective than any commercial diet she had tried in the past and acknowledged that it fitted into her day-to-day life much better than any of them.

Kate told me that the most difficult thing for her was getting used to eating vegetables, but this did get easier – easy in fact. She saw vegetables in a different light to how she had before, and didn't dismiss them out of hand. She tried them and enjoyed them. Her previous dislike of them had been based on what she imagined rather than experience. Her success with vegetables opened her mind to try other food she had previously dismissed, such as salmon and other fish, which again she found she enjoyed. Previous prejudices against certain foods had been based on faulty thinking.

I wanted Kate to think of moving forward into the future. I wanted her to envisage what her lifestyle was going to be like from now on, to ensure that she continued to achieve her desired goals. She said she intended to eat healthily, focus on portion control and frequently imagine herself as slim, sexy and gorgeous. I asked her what she thought the key to success was. Her answer? 'Don't give any shit excuses for being fat; it's up to you what you make of yourself, no one else. Ask yourself what you want to get out of this.' I was impressed – Life Bitch or what? Kate was enthused to share her new passionate approach to life with others – in fact, with everyone.

I also wanted to know how Kate would cope without my presence in her life, how she felt about going it alone. She was firmly of the belief that she would carry on the programme without difficulty, that she had the determination. She had the support of her family (her mum had also lost weight and was improving her fitness by joining Kate on her walks). Kate felt that one big motivating factor for her was for people to notice her as a slim, sexy woman. A real motivator would be her ability to turn men's heads and feel sexy in herself. Kate needed to imagine this end result, to see it, feel it and be it. I believed that this could happen; the process had already started. Kate agreed. She told me that, with her weight loss, she had been encouraged to go out in a sexy top, something she hadn't done for a long, long time. She was able to admire her curves, she saw that others noticed her, she felt sexy.

A key to Kate's continued success would be to keep seeing herself as she wanted to be. My advice to Kate was to continue to look at the repulsive picture of herself regularly and balance this with the picture in her mind of the end result, of herself as a head-turner. I knew she'd become a winner, who was proud to show off her new figure.

Sandra

What can I say about Sandra? She was a star. Following her progress on my programme, I knew I had found a Life Bitch Model of Excellence! All my participants did well and faced their challenges, all had a different story to tell of their progress and the changes they had made in their lives, but it was clear to me that, amidst all of this success, Sandra was the one who had grown the most. It was wonderful to witness. When I told her she was my Life Bitch Role Model of Excellence for the Midlands, she leapt from her seat and cried with joy. She was living proof that anything was possible in just a three-week period.

Sandra had lost 16 pounds, going from 15 stone 5 pounds to 14 stone 3 pounds.

She said that her biggest motivator had been my belief in her, which in turn had help foster her self-belief. Sandra had found that it was mainly the use of self-hypnosis and positive self-talk – done on a daily basis – that was the key to her success. She was very much focused on herself and the goal she desired. She discovered that it wasn't just about how she looked, but also how she felt about herself. She told me that she often used to think that others were thinking negative things about her, which meant that she had negative thoughts about herself. She said that this was no longer the case. In the three weeks of the programme, using the power of her mind to take control of two areas of her life – eating and exercise – she had affected much more profound changes than simply acquiring a slimmer, healthier body. No longer did she perceive herself in a poor light and her concerns about what others were thinking had gone. Sandra's sense of self had blossomed into something wonderful. All in three weeks! I was so proud of her, so impressed.

How easy or hard had she found the programme? Easy – yes. Hard – not at all. Once she had organised herself and planned her menus and her walking sessions, she found that the programme became very natural. The planning put her in control of these areas of her life.

She designated her own storage place for her food and enjoyed planning menus. She ate healthily – more fish, fresh vegetables, reasonable portions. She experienced no cravings or hunger, except for further success. She admitted that perhaps there had been a couple of difficulties. She had begun drinking lots of water – her recommended eight glasses a day – and she was finding that on her walks she often needed the loo. So how did she solve this? She planned the routes of her walks so that she could have loo breaks. Eventually, as Sandra's body became accustomed to taking in this extra liquid, this would no longer be an inconvenience. Also, at the start, she had found herself out of breath after walking. This didn't happen anymore and after each walk she felt energised, not knackered.

Three weeks had changed Sandra's habits, and this in turn had changed her life. I had inspired Sandra and she now had confidence in herself, something that she was willing to pass on to others.

I asked Sandra what it felt like to be a role model, an example to others, and she replied that she was so proud of herself. I wondered what she would reply to someone who said that changing your life in this way was too hard. Her answer? 'No it's not. You can do anything!'

Sandra had appreciated my support throughout the three weeks of the programme, although she did find my manner a bit scary to start with. But I had made her think. I had made her use her mind and helped her drill constructive messages into her head. From my first meeting with Sandra, I knew she could succeed the Life Bitch way. I saw beyond the anxiety, the fuss, the Drama Queen in her.

As my support and belief in Sandra had been especially important to her, I worried about how she would cope once I withdrew some of my contact. Talking to her about this, I was reassured. She said she felt very focused and was convinced she would keep up her new lifestyle and achieve her goal. Her big motivator was to picture herself looking good in jeans and brown boots. I was in no doubt she would do it. I observed that when I had first met Sandra, she hid her body, but now, although she still did this to some degree, it was now much less marked.

Sandra was proof that life can begin at 56 – for her it had.

One more story

There is one further programme participant that I really want to tell you about – Lisa.

Lisa is 45 years old. She has five kids, ranging in age from 27 to nine months, and one grandchild. If that isn't enough, she also has a part-time job as a senior secretary.

Unlike the other participants, Lisa, at 12 stone 7 pounds, wasn't massively overweight.

If anyone had excuses for not taking action, Lisa did: a large family, a demanding job and not being too obviously overweight. It would have been so easy for her to complain that she couldn't meet the requirements of my programme, that she couldn't find time to exercise or plan better meals, that her focus should be wholly on her family and not herself, that she wasn't too bad anyway. This was not Lisa's attitude though. She truly is an inspiration to those of us who can find reason after reason for not looking after ourselves.

Life Bitch

Lisa wanted to lose weight and get fitter. My advert for the Life Bitch programme caught her eye. She'd tried diets before and failed, but being part of my no-nonsense programme appealed to her. She sent me an email saying she needed a kick up the backside, that she'd lost her motivation somewhere along the way, and asking if I could help.

When I met her, she said she felt that she was always fighting to keep her weight down. She'd tried all the diets and now wanted something that would put her in control again.

I want to share Lisa's experience with you because, like many people, she only had a relatively small amount of weight to lose. I do know that it can be just as big a challenge for those people with a little to lose as those who literally have mountains to shift. Lisa rose to that challenge, and in the three weeks of the programme went from 12 stone 7 pounds to 11 stone 7 pounds.

I wanted to know how my Life Bitch programme had worked in her case. She said that the key for her had been to install positive affirmations in her mind. She already knew the facts about food and exercise – she clearly understood what she ought to eat, what she ought to do – but she needed to actively take steps to engage her mind in the process. I asked her if it had been easy to find time to fit in regular self-hypnosis, menu planning and walking. Lisa had realised that there is always time if you really want to do something.

Lisa was prepared to take full control of her life, which in her case was not easy. I remember visiting her house to find a

Brummie version of the Waltons – so many people calling on her time, so much activity going on all around. 'Quiet, John Boy! I'm doing self-hypnosis!' I have to conclude that she's an excellent role model to all those people who say that having kids makes it hard to effect changes.

One thing that Lisa did was to initially concentrate on *her* eating habits. She didn't try to change her family's habits at the same time. She fed the kids what they had been used to at the start, introducing healthy changes slowly and imperceptibly, in order to avoid unnecessary battles. She had to focus on her own needs first. For example, Lisa would cook a pasta bake for the kids and make a mixed-bean salad for herself. She would then give the children a little bit of the salad and encourage them to try it with her. By slowly introducing new foods to them and eating her own healthy meals in front of them, her kids soon began to enjoy the same meals she was eating.

At the end of the three-week programme Lisa had changed her habits. She knew she was in control. She was surprised how easy she had found the programme. In particular, she enjoyed making exercise part of her life – she's even joined a gym.

Lisa also reported other benefits that she hadn't anticipated. She:

✓ had more confidence

✓ had more choice of clothes

Life Bitch

- ✓ walked tall
- ✓ felt more relaxed
- ✓ had more energy
- ✓ slept better

Be a Life Bitch in three weeks

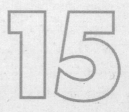

What follows is an example of a Life Bitch three-week plan. Use this plan for reference, to give you some sound ideas of how to construct your own Life Bitch weight-control strategy.

Week 1

Day 1

Make an appointment with your doctor to check out your ideal weight and suitability for gentle, progressive exercise such as walking, climbing stairs and swimming. Do not carry out what follows in this suggested programme unless you have confirmed this with your doctor or if you suffer from clinical depression or epilepsy.

When you get the green light, you have no lazy, fat-headed excuses not to start the Life Bitch programme.

This is a new start, so first of all go and take a cold shower. Allow the chill of the water to awaken your mind to what you are going to become; at last, a move away from being a true porky. As you take this shower, give yourself a firm talking to as you soap up the cellulite. If you find yourself a little tearful, let it all out; these are tears of realisation because you have had one hell of a wake-up call from your Life Bitch.

Tell yourself that things may not have worked out in the past, but at last you have found someone that doesn't wrap it up in cotton wool, someone who is going to ensure that you keep your arse on the wagon. Let's face it, if you fell off now you may bounce on those over-ample buttocks, but how long would it take you to get back on it? You're so unfit, you'd never catch up. In other words, chain yourself to the Life Bitch wagon.

Now go downstairs and throw out the crap foods. You already know what this means, so just do it. Once you've done this, pop down to the local supermarket and buy some healthy goodies, using your common sense. Ditch the pork scratchings in favour of raw vegetable sticks and low-fat hummus; dunk the doughnuts into the bin and get a punnet of fresh strawberries instead. You know the score.

When you get home, plan creative menus for three weeks as described on pages 239–51.

Day 2

Today you are going to go out and buy a couple of items of clothing in a smaller size than the tents you currently wear. However, please remember that I have no time for attention-seeking, size-zero divas, so keep it realistic. Buy something that is going to make you look and feel like a true sex bomb.

When you go to the counter to buy these clothes, look the assistant in the eye and tell him or her that these clothes are for you because you are a Life Bitch role model, someone who has got bags of oomph and determination to achieve a successful weight loss outcome. This is really important because you are already mentally becoming conditioned to naturally get off your arse to lose the saddlebags you carry round.

In the evening, go for a gentle 45-minute walk somewhere you'll feel relaxed and uplifted. Breathe in some fresh air and pay attention to the excess fat wobbling – every bit of wobbling means an extra bit of calorie busting. Smile as you walk and if you find yourself start to whinge, just shut up. Consciously tell yourself that you are going to increase your speed of walking and the distance you go and picture the fat dropping off onto the pavement.

Day 3

It is time to go and dig the photo album out of the loft or garage. Select one of the most disgusting, slob-like photographs you have of yourself and pin it on the fridge. Make this the picture that you are embarrassed to look at, the picture that, when you're showing your album to friends, is the one you quickly grab and say, 'You can't look at that one.'

Keep this nasty picture of you stuck firmly to the fridge door for the duration of your Life Bitch success journey. Each day, as you look at that picture, allow the utter revulsion to flow through your mind. When friends and family come to visit, ask them to look at the picture and ask them what they really think of it. Let them know that the elephant in the picture is the old you and it represents a phase in your life when you were simply a greedy-guts.

In the evening, take another 45-minute walk, but this time take a different route to show yourself that you really are going in a new, positive direction.

Days 4–7

Place your affirmations, as described on page 53, where they can be easily seen – on your wardrobe door, in the loo, in your car and so on.

These messages will drip-feed into your mind every day, ensuring that your success habits become more and more natural and deeply embedded into your unconscious mind.

> To put it simply: get rid of the garbage that blocks your life-change and welcome in clean, pristine, positive messages.

You are literally dumping out the rubbish and making room for something new. Each day, in your relaxed alpha state, affirm to yourself your positive life messages. Let them become an integral part of you. Up your game, because by now you are feeling really positive, and each evening take a 60-minute walk.

Week 2

Day 1

By now, you should already have lost some weight. If you haven't, then you haven't carried out the plan properly and have been stupid and lazy. So either start again on the Life Bitch path or stay fat.

If you *have* lost weight, then celebrate with a Life Bitch menu of top-class fruit, vegetables and a glass of high-quality wine. Then go for a refreshing and calorie-burning 60-minute walk and smile like a real winner. Think about the journey that you have come on so far. You've accepted that you were a loser in the past, but have moved on by ditching the bad habits and garbage food and making the life changes needed to be a Life Bitch winner.

On the walk, treat yourself to a bunch of flowers and when you buy them, explain to the assistant why you are buying them. Let them know you are a Life Bitch winner and what that means to you.

You know what to eat to be slim now – common-sense, low-fat, natural, fresh food and smaller helpings. Keep up the good work!

Day 2

Go for an early-morning walk today for an hour. Get up nice and early to prove to yourself that you are committed to change and not scared of the challenge.

Practise some visualisation of the successful outcome you are going to have. Picture yourself walking tall with a big smile on your face, wearing the outfit you've dreamt of wearing for years. This is a defined vision of you looking sexy and slender. Go for it!

Days 3–5

On these days, I want you to leap out of bed early and go on a 60-minute walk. After each walk, take a shower and sing out loud. Yes, sing. Don't worry if you are out of tune. I want you to sing loudly a song that gives you energy and makes you feel like a winner. Run your hands down your body and enjoy the feeling of success you get out of knowing that you are achieving your life goal of weight loss. When you get out of the shower, gently stretch your body and smile as widely as possible, saying the words, 'At last I am in control of my weight and am melting away the fat daily.' It has taken a lot of grit and determination to get where you are now and you damn well should start appreciating yourself.

When it comes to eating, notice how you fill up a bit quicker with every mouthful of food. That's simply because your stomach is shrinking, and so is the desire to stuff your face like you used to do.

Day 6

Today, think about the pathetic excuses you used to make – 'I'll start losing weight tomorrow,' 'I'm happy being fat' and so on. Write them down, look at them and then rip up the paper into as many tiny little pieces as possible. Throw them in the toilet, because that is where they belong, then pee on them. As you pee, realise that those stupid excuses used by fat people are going to be flushed away forever. This might sound unpleasant, but your mind is going to remember this process and what you felt when you did it. It is even better if you can do a number two on them as well before you flush. Get rid of the crap with the crap!

Day 7

Some time today, I want you to clean your home while playing your favourite music and dance yourself dizzy at the same time. Imagine yourself with your new shape as you dance – you'll enjoy the experience and burn calories.

Today is treat day, so go out and buy yourself something special. Maybe it is time to buy a new belt a couple of inches smaller or some new sexy underwear. You and I both know you are going to be irresistible now that you have chosen a new lifestyle. If you're feeling flush, buy a digital camera to record the new you and proudly fire off the pictures to your nearest and dearest.

Week 3

Day 1

By now, you have more than likely increased your energy levels, so step up the speed of your daily walking. If you are in any doubt about your ability to do this, then check things out with your doctor. I want you to step up the speed so that the sweat runs down your body. Imagine the sweat as fat literally melting from you because it really is.

You will, by now, be starting to feel, bodily and mentally, that your daily exercise is a pleasure, not a chore or a challenge, and it will be giving you a natural buzz. It has replaced the highs you sought through chocolate and junk food, and now you feel just fantastic.

Day 2

Today it is time for more mental, as well as physical, exercise. I want you to go into your mental 'motivation room' and talk to the part of your mind responsible for controlling your weight. Thank it, applaud it and ask it to carry on supporting you. Then affirm in your mind once again how fantastic it feels to be in control, unlike the other whingers who complain that they can't lose weight.

In the evening, go on another sweat-inducing walk. Go as fast as you can and try and sweat so much that you really stink when you get home. Let this be the odour of your success and a reminder of your journey so far.

Day 3

Today you are not going to be politically correct. I want you to go out of your way to really observe fat people stuffing their faces. Let this sickening sight repulse you. You'll find them in the fast-food outlets, shovelling fat and sugar down their gullets. You are not like those people now because you have shed pound after pound and don't get turned on by junk food anymore.

That's simply because you are strong and in control. Remember that it is the process of binge eating you are being repulsed by and not the people themselves. To help yourself feel that you are in the right, remember that we as a nation have collectively become the lardarses of Europe.

Day 4

You are now becoming so in control that you can take down some of the affirmations you've placed around the house and put them away somewhere safe. However, keep the picture of yourself on the fridge for a good few weeks yet, as we need that repulsion to stay firmly in your mind. As you take the affirmations down, I want you to mentally note that you are doing this because you have regained control over your eating habits, exercise and weight. Your life is now firmly on the right track.

As soon as you have done this, go out for a walk, smiling, skipping and, of course, sweating. The time has come for a celebration, so while you are on the walk, I want you to think of who you are going to invite to a dinner party you will be holding on day seven. Imagine the healthy meal you'll surprise them with and the compliments they will give you when they see the new, slimmer you.

Day 5

Come on, get out of bed and go for an early walk. If possible, choose a route that takes you to the top of a hill, where you can see for miles, and believe that the Life Bitch journey has taken you to a new height of control over your destiny. Feel the joy.

When you get home, contact your day-seven dinner guests. Invite as many or as few as you like. You may want to invite a couple of fatty friends, so they can see just how in control you are and what an inspiration you have become as a Life Bitch role model.

When you have done this, start to plan your Life Bitch menu. Remember: no crap foods. You are setting the example to yourself and your friends.

Day 6

Today, get your arse out of bed and immediately read out loud the Life Bitch pledge for long-term commitment, as set out below:

- I am a Life Bitch winner
- I have lost weight and will keep it off

! I will never go back to being the ashamed fat lump I used to be

! I love my new-found energy and lust for life

! I will always be a Life Bitch role model

Then go out for your morning walk. On the walk, think about how the Life Bitch way has worked for you. You haven't needed someone telling you what to eat — you have used your common sense. 'Diet' is a banned word; never tell people you have been losing weight on a diet.

Have a look at the Life Bitch website www.lifebitch.com to remind yourself that you are part of the Life Bitch army who are doing it for themselves. Maybe even drop the Life Bitch an email, sharing with him your success. Walk tall and sexy today. Gosh, you are becoming a flirt, aren't you? Good for you, you've earned it!

Day 7

It's party time!

Prepare for the party. Write out your healthy menu and display it on the table. Have some wine, but show how in control you are. Explain how fantastic you feel and that being a fat, lazy sod is no longer for you.

Show your friends that picture you never wanted others to see along with a new snap of you in something sexy and bewitching.

Life Bitch

Tell your guests that you are a Life Bitch and that you no longer accept that your future is being a fat, weak slob. Explain that you found it within yourself to change the course of your life and become a Life Bitch winner. Share a bottle of champagne with your friends and toast your future as a Life Bitch role model.

Getting it off and 16 keeping it off

You've seen the success of just four of my clients, who are living proof that the Life Bitch way works. You too can follow in their footsteps. By employing my methods you can get rid of that behemoth bottom, those titan tits, those hippo hips.

Getting it off

So what's the secret of getting the fat off and creating a fabulous body for yourself? It's simple: just take note of following seven points, and then DO them.

1 Stop going on about being too fat and the need to lose weight. Stop talking about it. Apart from making you boring, the more you talk rather than do, the more you try to analyse the problem, the more difficult this simple issue will seem. Losing weight isn't rocket science; it isn't like you're working out the meaning of life. It's easy. Accept it. Overcomplicating this problem is simply your way of excusing yourself from taking action.

2 Follow my advice in Chapters 2 to 6. Get motivated and, crucially, start to use my self–hypnosis techniques on a daily basis. I cannot stress enough how important this aspect of the Life Bitch programme is. If you don't do it, the programme won't work.

3 Keep in your mind the thought that fat is repulsive.

Try this now: run your hands down your figure and imagine how much of a turn off it would be to a lover to feel your ripples, wobbles and waves.

4 Make sure that you plan your menus and let them guide you when you shop for your weekly groceries. Take a shopping list with you and stick to it. Use your common sense and eat what you know is good for you. You don't need gimmicky diets or the media to tell you what you already know. Keep your menus simple and forget about the latest complicated recipes.

5 When friends and family members tempt you with something you know you shouldn't eat, avoid saying, 'No, I'm on a diet.' Remember: diet is a dirty word! Instead say, 'No, thanks. I don't want to be a fat pig.' If the person offering you the extra helping of pie or second glass of wine is a fat pig themselves and you feel this is too harsh, simply say, 'No, thanks. I want to be slim and nothing will stop me being that.' But consider sticking to the first reply – you might convert them to the Life Bitch way!

6 Look at the fat people you come across day to day and remind yourself just how lazy they are. The only exercise they probably do is lifting a knife and fork. Don't be like them. In other words, get off your backside and start moving!

7 Finally accept you have joined project JFDI. JUST F***ING DO IT!

If you've stuck with the book so far, I have every faith in you. I know you can start to shift that excess weight and let the fabulous you start to emerge.

Keeping it off

People often start their journey to weight loss well and then start to pile it back on, especially when the novelty has worn off.

Life Bitch

Making the changes permanent is down to you. Remember that becoming fat again is going to make you less attractive, lower your confidence and might well lead to an earlier death. Surely this makes a healthier lifestyle an obvious choice?

Follow the advice in this book or revert back to boring other people with your story about how much weight you once lost, but how you put it back on again and now you want to lose that weight again but there's never the time to do it. Do you honestly think anybody gives a toss that you want to lose weight for the holidays or that you'll start a weight-loss programme after Christmas? I doubt it. No, actually I don't – I know it.

So what's the secret of keeping the weight off?

1 If you carry out the self-hypnosis techniques on pages 77–88, your unconscious mind will make weight control a natural part of everyday living. If you haven't done the mind exercises, then it won't. Again, I must stress the importance of this mind work; it is fundamental to the Life Bitch programme.

2 As you start to lose weight, your stomach will shrink and you will find portion control easier. You will find it difficult to shovel in what you used to do; you'll wonder how you ever managed it.

3 Affirm personal control. When you go shopping, be proud you are now an arse-kicking Life Bitch who is buying clothes in smaller sizes. Continue to notice the fatties around you, lunging towards the doughnuts. Be repulsed and refuse to join that club again.

4 Run your hands down your body and feel how different it is now. Delight in the experience of being svelte, sexy and flirty. If losing weight brought new opportunities such as a love affair or better sex with your partner, enjoy it, but remember that the joy of sex will be diminished if he or she begins to notice that you're heavier when you're on top.

The slimmer's dream

I call this simple 'mind map' the slimmer's dream. It will help you picture the journey you're on and stick to it.

'As a successful slimmer, I see weight loss as being…'

Specific: I eat slowly, smile as I take pride in my new control, make confident eye contact, wear smaller-sized clothes, swagger proudly when I walk, tell people of my success, say 'No, thank you' to crap food, ask for smaller portions, feel in control, confident and sexy and am a bit of a flirt at times.

Measurable: I reach milestones, as defined in my vision of reaching my ideal target weight and dress size, mentally seeing that ultimate weight as reality right now.

Achievable: I believe it is possible. (If you have any doubts, shout out 'IT IS ACHIEVABLE!' and quit moaning.)

Realistic: I know it is common sense. Healthy foods are widely available and cheap and I'm armed with mind techniques that will boost my self-confidence and self-control.

Time-bound: My desired outcome will be achieved by... (Have a realistic date in mind, and bloody well make sure you do it by then.)

Don't forget to walk tall, be proud and to take control of your life right now.

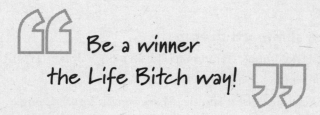

Be a winner
the Life Bitch way!

the
BITCH *list*

- Stop whining and just do it. Follow the advice in this book and the fat will melt away.
- Don't forget your self-hypnosis techniques. They are crucial to getting the weight off and, more importantly, keeping it off.
- Always keep the 'slimmer's dream' in mind.

Real life

Patricia contacted me and explained that she had an underactive thyroid and wanted to lose weight. She was 10 stones and 8 pounds and was desperate to get her weight down, as she had very high cholesterol and was worried she might have a heart attack. Her mother had died at 55 of heart failure, so you can imagine the anxiety she felt at being so flabby. Recently, she emailed me to thank me for the Life Bitch approach. She is now 8 stone 13 pounds, at a height of five feet four inches, and is obviously happier. What's more, she has taken up indoor rock climbing and has loads of energy.

Patricia is an inspiration to us all.

Green-eyed monsters

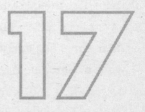

Once you start to shed those unwelcome pounds you will start to notice that people are treating you very differently. There will be those who welcome the new you wholeheartedly and unreservedly, those who are shocked and those who become edgy and fearful. The latter can be real problems for you. They are jealous that you look more attractive now and they might even go as far as trying to sabotage your Life Bitch programme and encourage you to pile on the lard again.

Be aware, in fact be very aware, of these green-eyed monsters. They are the vicious bacteria that will do everything they can to get you to stuff the crap nosh inside you again. As you now have new-found self-esteem, self-worth and a positive outlook on life you will find it easier to deal with these people. But let's think about how to avoid and/or deal with the typical green-eyed monsters.

Monster 1: your partner

It is quite natural for your partner to become insecure as a result of you looking slim and fabulous, so do your best to reassure them. Let them know that they are the one for you and that you have never felt so good about your relationship. Be there, give them time, be patient, but if they become so obsessed that they want to put you on a leash, then it may be time to put your foot down.

Explain that under no circumstances will you be the object of their obsessive possession. Stay strong and let them see just how loyal you are to the relationship. Don't stop showing off your new, cute arse in the fashions that you have always wanted to wear – there is nothing wrong with that – but let them see that you always come home to them and that they are what matters to you. If, however, their possessive attitude continues and they continue to encourage you to eat extra roasties or drink more wine, then you need to take stock of your relationship.

You have moved on with your life and opened up a completely new chapter. Your partner has to be able to cope with this. If they can't, then perhaps you need to move on from them. Think about the reasons why you were an overweight loser. Did your partner hold you back? Did they drain you of motivation, add extra stress to your life and make you feel useless? If the answer is yes, then perhaps it is time to ditch them.

Monster 2: your best friend

Your best mate sees you losing the flab. You dance better than she does when you're on a night out, men give you the eye more than her and she is becoming insecure every time you dare to speak to her man. Of course, you want to keep her as your best friend. After all, she has supported you when you were a big bird and you ate late-night curries together, gorged on cream cakes when times got tough and shared a big tub of ice cream as you watched your favourite movie together.

If you find yourself with a friend like this, make sure you initially assure her that she is still your best mate and that if she wants to follow your lead, you will be there for her all the way. Don't get into an argument if she claims you are eyeing up her bloke now that you have lost the weight – this is pointless and a waste of precious time and energy.

Say positive things to your friend like, 'You are looking fantastic and those leggings really look good on you now that you have lost a few pounds' or 'Thanks for stopping me from scoffing those biscuits with my coffee.' Comment on what they are great at, even if it's not getting off their fat arse and losing some weight. Look like you mean it and make sure you sound excited, interested and happy. If all fails and your friend remains a miserable, jealous pain in the arse, get rid of them and make some new mates.

Let's face it, now that you are reborn, making friends has never been easier. People want to get to know you and are inviting you to social events a hell of a lot more. So don't feel that you will be alone if you are forced to give the two-fingered salute to a so-called 'best friend'. Celebrate, because you don't have time for people who are emotional drains anymore.

Your new friends will see you as the butterfly who has cracked the fat cocoon that held you back and will treat you as you should be – with respect, love and friendship.

Monster 3: your colleagues

Your workmates will either cheer or boo your successful trip to Life Bitch triumph. As you drop the pounds, you will be treated differently by the boss, the customers and the staff. You may well find yourself becoming known as the bit of stuff in the department because you look so good! Don't be surprised if phone numbers are offered and the person you once dreamt of getting it on with asks you out to dinner.

But beware of the colleagues who craftily pop a Twix on your desk with morning coffee or place a piece of chocolate cake on your desk because it's someone's birthday. If this happens, remember your Life Bitch basics and do some self-affirmation: you have become who you want to be and you are not going to sneak a chocolate biscuit or three, you love what you have become and you are in control, etc.

If you feel that you are about to give in to temptation, see that big red stop sign. When you see and smell that chocolate cake, engage your brain and say, 'I've gone off cake.' Just say 'no'!

Don't become too cocky as you lose the weight and start to feel fabulous, but do stay strong. Be friendly and positive with your colleagues, but let it be known that nothing will take your focus off the Life Bitch course now. Take your lunch into work and if people offer to take you out, be assertive and tell them you are too busy. If a jealous workmate tries to coax you out to have a good chat over a BLT sandwich and fries, stand tall and politely refuse, unless you are sure that healthy options will be available.

There will be plenty of people at your workplace who will be bowled over by your dramatic weight loss and new image and who will give you loads of positive feedback. Feel fantastic, because you have earned it.

Monster 4: your neighbour

Picture the scene. You have dropped a few dress sizes, feel fit and have a glam new look, while Plain Jane next door remains a few stone overweight and continues to wear those elastic-waisted tracksuit trousers. She sees you walking out to the car, head held high, proud, happy and looking like sex on legs. Because she is insecure, she stops calling you or popping round for a cup of tea (and, in her case, a packet of biscuits) and is distant when you bump into her.

Don't let it get to you. She probably has low self-esteem and blames her weight problem on some flimsy excuse that you know is just a silly escape hatch.

At first, try to keep the relationship friendly. Ask her round for a smoothie or make her feel special by asking her advice about something. Leave a copy of your Life Bitch journal out for her to see and encourage her to try it for herself. Maybe ask her to go walking with you, but if you do take it easy, as it may be the first time she's got off her arse and done a bit of exercise for years.

If all fails and the dismissive looks continue, the doorbell doesn't ring and she keeps her man away from you, then enough is enough. Let her go and leave her to remain the victim she seems to enjoy being. Remember: it's not your problem, it's hers.

Monster 5: your family

This is a hard one because your nearest and dearest should really have been supportive of your Life Bitch programme and overjoyed by your weight loss. However, you might have siblings, teenage kids, parents etc. who could do with shifting their own saddlebags, and seeing you succeed in this may trigger their jealousy.

It might be that you have a teenage daughter who is finding it hard to get the boy she wants because she is overweight, while you have found new love because of the new you. If she's showing signs of jealousy, be sensible and explain that you have achieved your life dream by shedding the fat. Tell her that you will help her to successfully lose weight through the Life Bitch programme. Above all, get her to understand that no one else can lose weight for her, but that she already has the motivation within her to succeed.

Perhaps your dad has let himself go around the middle and you have shared jokes in the past about your bulging tums. Now you have slimmed down, you think your dad is treating you differently and not cuddling you as much as he used to. This is a classic sign of insecurity. He needs to do something about it and he can, with your help. Sit down with him and tell him how you now feel as a Life Bitch role model. Discuss your new confidence and the joy you are experiencing because you are slimmer. Tell your dad you love him and want him to get on the Life Bitch programme. Let him know that his age is not an excuse not to lose weight and that he would be setting the younger people in the family a brilliant example by getting rid of the tum. He will respect you for being honest with him.

Although facing the jealousy caused by the new you and dealing with it can be difficult, it can also help with your long-term motivation. People are being jealous for one reason: they want to look and feel like you. Use this as something positive to keep fuelling your Life Bitch motivation. Even if someone is being horrible to you, smile, look into their eyes and say, 'I can help you to get slim and feel like you are on top of the world.'

the BITCH *list*

- Be patient with your partner and reassure them that you are still there for them, but if they continue to hold you back, it's time to take stock of the relationship.
- If your friends are unable to support you on your journey to a new, slimmer you, it's time to put your new-found confidence to good use and make some new ones.
- Keep an eye out for green-eyed monsters that try crafty tricks to get you to stuff crap food in your gob.
- Be a role model to your family and encourage them to join you on your journey.
- Be friendly and positive to all those around you, but stay strong!

Bitch be good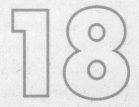

So you like being a role model for the Life Bitch army and you enjoy shouting about the new you and the self-control you have when it comes to sensible eating and exercise. I welcome you on board, but I want to make certain things clear as you champion our common cause. Being a Life Bitch isn't about shouting and bullying people into doing things they don't want to do. It's about providing strong, direct guidance to help move people away from a fat, sedentary lifestyle.

If, at the end of the day, people want to go week after week to a slimming club to talk about how 'naughty' they have been for sneaking a bar of chocolate because they were a bit down, then let them. These are the people who will remain stuck in the same rut, and, no matter how hard you try, you won't kick them out of it.

I know this isn't your style because you have chosen the Life Bitch way, but some people seem to live for the latest fad diet and slimming group. They are life's victims, who love being caught in this cycle of talk and no real action.

As a Life Bitch model of excellence, I actively encourage you to offer advice to friends and family about the practical things they can do to turn around their lazy minds, bubble-like figures and conditioned bad habits. But how you do this is really important. Being fair and assertive, rather than aggressive and undermining, is the key. It is the assertive style of Life Bitching that I want you to learn.

By assertive, I mean firmly leading your family and friends by positive examples, such as cutting out your dependency on takeaway meals and supermarket food deliveries. Tell people that you are leading a new lifestyle and be firm and confident when you encounter their natural resistance to change. If you are trying to change your family's habits, be fair with them; allow the occasional treat and give them goals to work with you on, like a family trip to your nearest theme park.

> Being an assertive Life Bitch isn't about always getting your own way and saying that others must adapt.

It is, at the end of the day, their choice. If they want to stay fat, then, short of muzzling them, there isn't much you can do. The assertive Life Bitch states clearly what she or he thinks should happen in a direct, firm manner and at the same time recognises that others may disagree.

To deal with disagreements, you will need to hone your negotiation skills, partly by using rewards and partly by realising that other people's ability and commitment to change their lifestyles may not be as great as yours. Stick to your guns and keep plugging away, and it will rub off on them. They will become more involved and start to do things the Life Bitch way.

How to be assertive the Life Bitch way

I want you to consider the following advice on being assertive:

- Being assertive is totally different from being aggressive. Aggressive Life Bitching is when you want to get your own way at all costs, ignoring the other person's point of view. If you ever feel this happening, take some deep breaths and calm down. If you can't, leave the room. Once you have relaxed, think negotiation

- Negotiation. Your family and friends are likely to have different values and priorities to you. Don't ride roughshod over them when you are trying to win them over to the Life Bitch way of thinking

❗ Use your brain and think about what will attract their support and commitment. For example, if your partner assumes you can't cook, won't cook and that's why you buy in processed ready-meals and takeaways, surprise them with a fail-safe, healthy meal that you have prepared from scratch. Enjoy their disbelief and pleasure when they find out this was all your own work, and tell them that they can look forward to more of the same. To take another example, motivate your kids to get active by spending whatever you can afford on some sports kit or equipment for them

Keep it simple and it will work.

❗ Clearly explain to your family and friends the actions that you want to take and what your goals are. Just binning all their favourite snacks without telling them first will piss them off royally. You need to involve them and get them to agree, however grudgingly, to support you on your journey

❗ Lead by example and pin up the pictures of you that were under lock and key before. Show your loved ones that you are determined to change your life and they will start to engage with you about it. This confidence to move things forward will inspire them as well as you

! Crucial to your role as an assertive Life Bitch is your
ability and desire to actively listen to the views of others.
You have got to appreciate and respect other points of
view, even if you disagree

When you have listened to what someone has to say, state what you think. Speak calmly and use the 'I' stance to emphasise this is your personal opinion. For example, you might say, 'I appreciate that you think it is harder to lose weight as you get older, but I consider this to be an escape hatch that people use to stay fat.' Demonstrate empathy by discussing in detail the reasons why they feel getting older blocks weight loss and then conclude the conversation with your point of view. For example, 'I appreciate that you think it is harder to lose weight as you get older because you can't exercise as much and your metabolism has slowed down, but I still think this isn't a valid excuse, as exercise can be as gentle as walking for half an hour, doing a bit of gardening or getting off the bus a stop or two early, and by doing this you will speed up your metabolism. Therefore, I would always advise people to rid themselves of excuses and put in some work to get slim.'

Proactive Life Bitching

There will be plenty of opportunities for you to evangelise about the Life Bitch approach to weight loss, and I would like you to seize them. You will get others to take control of their weight and it will make you feel brilliant.

Your achievement needs to be shouted from the rooftops, and if this can benefit others, then it is all good stuff. Walk tall, ooze confidence and tell people why the Life Bitch is working for you.

Let me give you some tips to help you become a proactive Life Bitch.

1 Offer advice on how people can programme their minds. Describe to them some of the techniques in this book. Point out the particular techniques that worked for you and motivated your mind to slim down naturally.

2 Offer to give them a written list of the typical excuses we use for not losing weight. Then offer a Life Bitch response to each.

3 Recommend some initial steps to take, such as buying a piece of clothing a couple of sizes smaller and hanging it in plain sight at home or the ritual of throwing out the junk food/processed food with the trash.

4 Show your friends how to design a Life Bitch menu. Tell them which ones worked for you. Even better, invite them over for a Life Bitch meal you have prepared using fresh, exciting and healthy ingredients.

5 Teach your friends and family to say 'f**k off' to crap food. Explain to them how you manage to resist too many portions of fish and chips or a heart-stopping burger.

6 Share with others the Life Bitch way to help kids be truly healthy in what they eat and how to get them to become more physically active.

7 Tell people that you are a Life Bitch who can identify the 'drains' that keep holding you back. Give them examples of unhelpful comments like, 'You don't need to lose any weight,' 'What's wrong with carrying a few extra pounds?' or 'It's Friday – let your hair down and have a cake.' Challenge them to say 'no' to anything that they don't want to eat.

8 Share with others the support and direction that you have got by keeping a Life Bitch journal. Explain that being honest with themselves and remembering key techniques and affirmations by writing them down is vital to progressive, sustainable weight loss.

Now that you are aware of what it means to be a Life Bitch role model and how to conduct yourself, I want you to lose no time and start Life Bitching for the good of everyone. Get the word out and start to be an inspiration to those you love.

the BITCH list

- Concentrate on being assertive rather than aggressive.
- Hone your negotiation skills.
- Lead others by example.
- Try to empathise with people and never be rude or dismissive.
- Be a proactive Life Bitch and encourage others to join the programme by offering advice on the initial steps they should take.

A thin line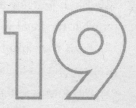

As the chapter title suggests, the issue of 'when is slim too slim' is a very tricky one; it is a thin line. There's constant media hype surrounding celebrities and models who are painfully thin. The problem is that one minute a glossy magazine is placing stick-thin people on a pedestal and the next minute they are saying that so-and-so has got too thin and has a problem. My advice is to step away from this debate and not let yourself be driven by the media when making life choices, especially when it comes to body image.

As your Life Bitch, I do not endorse trying to achieve a pencil-thin body. Yes, there are people out there who are naturally super-skinny or 'size zero', call it what you will. It is for that reason that I want to drum it into you that once your ideal weight has been achieved you should stick to it. You look great – enjoy it! Don't carry on shedding weight, so that you look unhealthy or worse.

You should have consulted your doctor before starting on this Life Bitch journey and therefore will have a professional opinion on what the ideal weight is for your gender, age and height. This has been the target and the reason for following the Life Bitch programme, so make sure you stick to it. I don't want any bullshit excuses for crossing the line.

How to avoid crossing the thin line

1 Stay grounded. You have harnessed control of your mind and body, but I want you to be grounded at all times and not abuse your new power. I want you to consciously monitor your thought patterns and if you hear yourself say 'Just a few more pounds' when you have hit your ideal weight, then picture that big red stop sign. You are not, in fact, in control anymore if you deliberately go under your ideal weight, and I certainly do not want you as one of the Life Bitch army.

2 Use your Life Bitch journal to track your progress to your ideal body weight and don't avoid logging your progress if you go below this weight, so that you can see it in black and white. In fact, record this in red, because you are starting to cross into a potentially dangerous zone.

3 Make yourself aware that people who are very thin don't actually look good. How many times have you heard people comment on how bony someone looks, that they could do with a good meal? Stick-thin and bony is not attractive. You might find it difficult to find adult clothes, and those that you do find will hang off you. Remind yourself of that, please. And I don't want to hear any bollocks about losing a bit extra now so you can go on a booze fest at the end of the month. That is a terrible attitude; you will be damaging your mind and body.

4 Remind yourself again that when you have hit your ideal weight, you can have the odd plate of fish and chips. Stay realistic and in control by reaffirming to yourself that you made the situation good under your own steam and that you now eat sensibly and exercise frequently, but that you also recognise that joining the size-zero clan is not for you and will never happen.

5 Keep visualising your ideal shape and notice that it is not bony and stick-thin. Make sure that you carry out this visualisation technique at least three times a day. This will then be firmly embedded in your unconscious mind and will protect you from crossing the line.

6 Avoid looking in magazines that portray 'their' ideal shape, as it's likely to be a skeletal one. The models that go on Operation Starvation look bloody awful. So get it right out of your head that you will look more attractive and pull new lovers if your bones are sticking out. Yes, you will be looked at, but for all the wrong reasons. Ditch the magazines and be proud to tell your friends that you don't take any notice of them anymore when they start discussing how thin the latest Hollywood stars look. Tell them you love the way you look and feel proud that you aren't following the pack.

7 You won't ever need to cross the line if you stick to the Life Bitch way of losing weight because it is the right way. You must exercise and eat regularly and correctly, and at all times keep weight loss in perspective. Never starve yourself or try to lose 30 pounds in a month. You know the score. It is common sense – around two or three pounds per week is healthy. Life Bitch winners are sensible, practical thinkers who use their minds not their emotions to make decisions about eating.

8 Working with your Life Bitch buddy will help you to keep it real and make sure you stay on target for your ideal body weight, not above or below it. They will be on hand to tell you if you have overstepped the mark.

9 Remember that you are a Life Bitch role model and going under your ideal weight sets a piss-poor example, especially to young people.

If you find yourself obsessing about losing more weight than you should, visit your GP because there are some real and present dangers to consider, as the following case study outlines.

Real life

I really want to highlight the point that becoming obsessive about your weight and body image can be fatal.

Ana Carolina Reston had been modelling since she was 13. When she died, aged 21, she weighed just six stone. Clinically, her death was due to the diet of apples and tomatoes she had been living on for months in a bid to stay crazily thin, which caused her kidneys to pack up. But you could say that her death was caused by the current obsession with models that are painfully and often unnaturally thin.

The five-foot-seven Brazilian spent the last three weeks of her life in hospital. Her death shows that designers are still using size-zero models who are clearly suffering from eating disorders, despite calls to stop using these girls because they encourage eating disorders in other young women. This is what really baffles me: why are unnaturally thin models and celebrities being encouraged to stay as they are?

The trend for size-zero models — equivalent to a British size four — began as a fad in Los Angeles and Ana Carolina Reston's case is not an isolated one.

If you start to cross that thin line we have spoken about, then you've got to be aware that the consequences can be terrible. I want you to look at your fat photographs and then take a look at yourself now. Understand how fantastic you look at your healthy, ideal weight. Don't take it any further. You are my Life Bitch role model and I am proud of you, so stay that way!

the BITCH list

- Don't be driven by the media when it comes to body image.
- Do not go beyond your ideal weight. Stay in control.
- Remember that stick-thin bodies are not attractive to the majority of the population.
- Keep visualising your ideal shape, and notice that it is not size zero.
- Talk to your Life Bitch buddy about not crossing the line and help each other to keep it real.
- If you are ever concerned visit your GP.

Life begins at page 231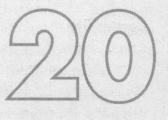

Y ou are only permitted to read this final chapter if you have made it. By 'made it' I don't necessarily mean hit your ideal target weight just yet. 'Made it' means that you have turned around your life and become a champion of weight control the Life Bitch way. You have developed a mindset that has given you conscious control over your eating habits, recognised that it isn't difficult to lose weight and have at last ditched the excuses and become more motivated to take personal responsibility. You have left the 'blame culture' behind, and I am proud of you.

Among other things, your new life begins when you can run your hands around your backside and appreciate how cute it's becoming, walk into a clothes store and slip easily into the outfit of your choice and sit confidently in the seat you once had to squash into.

Let's take a little time to look at what life has become for you and the possibilities that are now beginning to open up.

Career life

Fatism is alive and well in the workplace, whether we like it or not. I read recently that *Personnel Today*'s February 2007 survey of 2,603 HR professionals found that almost half believe obesity negatively affects employee output. More concerning was the fact that 93 per cent of respondents said they would hire a 'normal weight' applicant as opposed to an obese one if they were identically qualified. Believe it or not, the immediate assumption made by most people who are a normal body weight is that people who are obese are lazy because they have allowed their bodies to get out of condition. Like it or not, this is a fact of life, and you never want to go back there.

Now new doors will begin to open for you as you glide into that interview with a slimmed-down frame, smart appearance and inner and outer confidence. You look like a quality, go-getting product, rather than an under-confident snail that may let the team down. It's time to consider what you really want to do with your career. You are feeling better about yourself, so now may be the time to consider a change of direction. Remember that it isn't unusual to have four careers in one lifetime these days, so go do it if it feels right.

If you work in a call centre because you couldn't bear the thought of people seeing you in the flesh, then maybe it's time to consider putting your new confidence to good use. It could be that you always thought you would be a brilliant salesperson if your body language hadn't always let you down because you were fat, or that a career in PR beckons because you now look the part of a really confident communicator. The possibilities have become almost boundless. So get out there and go for it!

Love life

Sex may now be firmly back on your menu, taking the place of those cream cakes, but I want to offer you a few words of caution.

Lovers may envy the change in you. If this is the case, start by reassuring them and tell them this is the real you and that you will be stronger together.

As for your sex life, let those bedroom activities get steamy and burn even more calories than your power-walking. You, my dear, can keep the lights switched on, look at yourself in the mirrors on the ceiling and jump on top without worrying about suffocating the poor partner beneath you.

My clients report time and time again that sex has never been so good since dropping their dress or waist sizes. In fact, they claim that they demand more and more, and so do their lovers. Your appeal is hotting up by the day, so enjoy it! Keep the *Karma Sutra* by the bed and try some new positions.

If you are single, be fussier and date only those that turn your head and stimulate your mind. Don't be frightened to let your new-found confidence shine. Draw up a shortlist and test them out!

Your life

Confidence, large helpings of self-esteem and increased physical fitness are just a few of the new things in your life. So many doors will now open to you on the social scene. I remember one client explaining that she wanted to go and see *Mama Mia!* in London, but was so afraid that she wouldn't fit into the theatre seat. She was also aware that her breathing was strained and loud due to her weight and was worried that this might annoy those sitting near her.

No fear for you! This is the time for partying, socialising and doing all the things you wanted to do when you were at home stuck in your role of couch potato. Perhaps it's time to join the local football or netball team and rediscover a sport that used to be a passion but which you had to drop when you became an unfit blob. Or maybe you could have a go at line dancing or belly dancing, both of which can be a real hoot. The latter would previously have been a real no no, openly showing off all those flabby folds, but now you can hold your head high and shake it with the best of them.

Family life

Being involved with the family has to be one of the greatest satisfactions for parents and those of you who are close to kids. To be able to see your children following in your footsteps like true winners, controlling their weight, is fantastic.

You can be so proud of yourself for saying enough is enough and taking on Life Bitch actions to nurture a lifestyle change. If the kids were fat and have become, or are becoming, slimmer, then it is less likely they will be bullied at school and they will begin to enjoy significant health benefits. Your children, and those who see you as a role model, will thank you for showing them that life doesn't have to be dictated by other people and circumstances. They can be masters of their futures, as you are.

As a family, life will certainly become loads more fun. You are now able to play actively together without becoming out of puff and can eat in a restaurant without being ridiculed.

I am so happy that you can now show your family that a sensible approach to eating and exercise can be fun and one hell of an achievement and that they have supported you and joined you on your journey.

Longer life

Increased longevity of life is a big win for all my Life Bitch role models. Yes, you can enjoy your new life more fully, but, even better, you have a longer life in front of you to savour.

Life Bitch

Above all, by losing this excess fat you are now someone that can take advantage of the benefits that this new lease of life delivers. In all probability it has been extended by a considerable amount, probably years. You have made it, and I am celebrating this with you. Once upon a time this might have seemed impossible, but your Life Bitch believed in you and now you can believe in yourself.

the **BITCH** *list*

- You've done it, tiger, so celebrate!
- Is it time for a career change? Now you have new-found confidence, do some research and go out and get the job you've always wanted.
- If you are after a new relationship, be choosy. Carry out a good M.O.T assessment on any potential dates.
- You now have plenty of energy, so take up new hobbies and rediscover old passions.
- Keep encouraging and motivating your family.
- Enjoy your longer life!

Final thoughts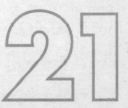

So there you have it. My route to success.

I've given you the tools, now it's up to you. My clients are living proof that the Life Bitch method works. You can't resist me. But it is down to you.

Come on, just do it. What have you got to lose other than unsightly excess flesh?

What you have to gain is: energy, control, pride, a fabulous sexy body… I could go on and on.

 So what's stopping you?

Life Bitch

Remember this MEMO:

> **M**ind work
>
> **E**xercise
>
> **M**enus
>
> **O**h, don't you look fabulous!

You are a 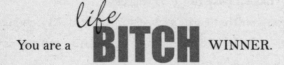 WINNER.

Appendix

The Life Bitch menu plans

Don't forget to drink at least eight glasses of water every day.

Sunday

Breakfast

Juicy selection of pineapple chunks, papaya, orange segments and banana slices

Glass of organic apple juice

Lunch

Spit-roasted herby chicken served with seasonal green vegetables
and sweet potato

Wholegrain scone with fresh strawberries

Fresh ground coffee or tea

Dinner

Leafy salad accompanied by a portion of poached salmon, dressed with a
mixture of light oil, balsamic vinegar and mustard

Monday

Breakfast

Crunchy granola accompanied by a perfectly ripened pear
Tea

Lunch

Tasty, freshly prepared wrap stuffed with crisp peppers, mushroom,
lettuce and tomato

Dinner

Grilled chicken fillet wrapped with lean bacon on a bed of rocket leaves,
accompanied by mangetout
Tangy assortment of mixed sorbet, sprinkled with crunchy almonds
Organic fruit juice

Tuesday

Breakfast

Creamy porridge with fresh blueberries
Glass of organic orange juice

Lunch

Piping-hot chunky vegetable soup
Wholemeal country roll

Dinner

Sizzling stir-fried onions, peppers, mushrooms, bean sprouts,
carrots and tofu enlivened with soy sauce
A selection of seasonal fruits

Wednesday

Breakfast

Banana, strawberry and raspberry blended into a smoothie
with some natural yogurt and honey

Lunch

Low-fat cheese, bacon and tomato sandwich, made with wholemeal bread

Dinner

Oven-roasted aubergine, accompanied by sweet potato and tomatoes
flavoured with balsamic vinegar and Mediterranean herbs
Mouth-watering assortment of pear, orange slices and passion fruit

Thursday

Breakfast

Hearty English breakfast of two rashers of lean, grilled bacon, a poached egg,
a grilled tomato, mushrooms and a slice of toast — dry or with low-fat spread
Tea

Lunch

Wholemeal roll of tuna and salad
Juicy blood orange with a little muscovado sugar

Dinner

Crispy-skinned jacket potato with cottage cheese,
accompanied by a spicy three-bean salad

Friday

Breakfast

Bran flakes drenched with ice-cold skimmed milk,
sprinkled with dried fruit and crunchy nuts
Glass of freshly squeezed orange juice

Lunch

Tender turkey salad with pine nuts and a low-fat orange and chilli dressing
Organic elderflower juice

Dinner
Medley of mouth-watering melon
Wholemeal pasta with mangetout, broccoli, mushroom, garlic and crème fraîche

Saturday

Breakfast
Two slices of wholemeal toast topped with honey
Tea

Lunch
Banana, strawberry and orange smoothie
Some of your favourite nuts and dried fruit

Dinner
Stir-fry of tender, lean beef strips, mushroom, bean sprouts
and garlic with soy sauce
Half-bottle of chilled white wine

Sunday

Breakfast
Homemade granola with natural yogurt
Glass of banana and orange juice

Lunch
Tray-roasted courgettes, tomatoes and mushrooms with a splash of soy sauce
and a sprinkle of dried chillli
Purée of apple and ginger with a dash of natural yogurt

Dinner
Skinny fish pie made without the cream and butter, but with plenty of
white fish, thick scalloped potatoes and parsley served with French beans

Monday

Breakfast
Favourite dried fruits e.g. apricots, apples and dates with some natural honey
Fresh mango juice

Lunch
Toasted wholemeal sandwich with tuna, olives and watercress
Pure fruit smoothie

Dinner
Grilled whole mackerel stuffed with sundried tomatoes (minus the oil)
Low-fat peach milkshake with fruity bits

Tuesday

Breakfast
Low-fat blueberry muffin
Glass of organic orange juice

Lunch
Small baked potato with mixed spicy bean filling
Small lemon sorbet

Dinner
Wild mushroom risotto with mushroom stock and a dash of Vermouth
Baked pear infused with natural vanilla

Wednesday

Breakfast
Toasted crumpets spread with Marmite (no butter)

Lunch
Tomato and feta salad with olives

Dinner
Salt-baked white fish served with a Thai salad of leaves, lime juice and red chilli
Fresh orange and pear salad soaked in fruit juice with a twist of Cointreau

Thursday

Breakfast
Scrambled eggs with a little smoked salmon and a slice of wholemeal toast

Lunch
Wholemeal roll filled with lean roast beef and horseradish sauce
Dried mixed fruits with a little natural yogurt

Dinner
Shredded chicken stir-fried with baby corn and oyster mushrooms
served with wholemeal noodles
Pineapple frozen yogurt

Friday

Breakfast
Boiled egg with wholemeal toast soldiers
Organic apple juice

Lunch
Chicken breast with a crunchy salad of carrots, cabbage and lettuce
Organic pear juice

Dinner

Lean minced beef in a classic chilli con carne with a little boiled rice

Fresh pineapple with a spinkle of brown sugar

Saturday

Breakfast

Two slices of wholemeal toast topped with honey

Tea

Lunch

Banana, strawberry and orange smoothie

Some of your favourite nuts and dried fruit

Dinner

Stir-fry of tender, lean beef strips, mushroom, bean sprouts and garlic

with soy sauce

Half-bottle of chilled white wine

Sunday

Breakfast

Poached egg on a wholemeal muffin

Glass of organic pineapple juice

Lunch

Grilled monkfish with coriander and lime dressing,
served with minted new potatoes
Meringue nest served with fresh mango
Tea

Dinner

Cottage cheese with a Thai salad of mixed leaves
with chilli and lemongrass dressing
Tea

Monday

Breakfast

Wholemeal toast with honey
Tea

Lunch

Mixed bean salad with wild rice and field mushrooms

Dinner

Smoked salmon served on soda bread with a green side salad
Strawberry frozen yogurt served with fresh strawberries
Glass of organic grape juice

Tuesday

Breakfast

Weetabix topped with low-fat natural yogurt and dried mixed berries
Glass of organic apple juice

Lunch

Homemade onion soup
Apple and orange segments drenched in orange juice

Dinner

Grilled chicken and green pepper kebabs served with low-fat yogurt mixed with
some mint and chilli and a green salad
Baked apple with cinnamon and sultanas

Wednesday

Breakfast

Grilled, lean bacon served with grilled tomatoes
Mint tea

Lunch

Cottage cheese and crunchy vegetables in a wholemeal wrap

Dinner

Wholemeal pasta with courgettes and tomatoes

Banana and strawberry smoothie

Thursday

Breakfast

Plain toasted bagel with low-fat cream cheese

Glass of freshly squeezed grapefruit juice

Lunch

Tuna salad with olives and balsamic vinegar

Tea

Dinner

Fresh asparagus wrapped with Parma ham, served with a small baked potato

Fresh orange and pineapple pieces with frozen coconut yogurt

Friday

Breakfast

Scrambled egg served on a wholemeal muffin

Glass of freshly squeezed orange juice

Lunch
Carrot, cumin and coriander soup with a wholemeal roll
Glass of organic apple juice

Dinner
Griddled tuna steak with tomatoes and aubergine
Low-fat coffee-flavoured frozen yogurt

Saturday

Breakfast
Banana pancakes
Coffee

Lunch
Orange, couscous and chick pea salad

Dinner
Grilled sea bass served with lime and spinach
Half-bottle of chilled white wine

The Life Bitch journal

I'd like you to start a Life Bitch journal as soon as you decide that you are going to accept the Life Bitch route to achieving your ideal body weight and maintaining it. I have come up with an outline of what you should include in your journal to start you off and as a daily reminder to keep you on track to becoming a Life Bitch role model.

Mirror mirror . . .

I want your Life Bitch journal to be truly honest from the word go and to be a place where you can purge harmful emotions and find strength to carry you through some of the hard times you will face.

To start with I need you to find the worst pictures you have of yourself, pictures that make you ashamed and sad about how overweight you have become. I want you to stick one of these into your journal as a reminder of where you are coming from. I also want you to write down the feelings that this image makes you feel and, as I said, be completely honest. Are they embarrassment, disgust, feelings of failure, loss of control? Write these feelings down at the beginning of your Life Bitch journal because they will help to motivate you from now on.

I don't want you to hop on and off the weight scales every day, but do record your current, puffed-up weight now, and alongside it record what your target, ideal weight is, as directed by your doctor or professional health advisor. Alongside the disgusting picture of you at your lardy-arsed peak, place a cut-out image of your ideal body shape.

You now have a clear picture in your Life Bitch journal and in your mind about where exactly you need get to in order to be a Life Bitch winner.

The next step is to record the hopes and fears that you have for your Life Bitch journey. I want you to list what achieving your ideal weight will mean to you. For example, you might decide that when you reach your ideal weight you will get married to your partner or start a family or find a new career, etc. You might also have reservations about the positive outcome of losing the weight, such as losing your emotional crutch (the junk food) or losing friends who can't stand to see the butterfly you have become. I want you to write these feelings down as well. These jottings will be an anchor for your motivation – you can read through your hopes and fears at any time to remind you what you are striving to achieve and that the fears are by far outweighed by the benefits.

Day by day

Here is a guide to the kinds of things you should record on a daily basis as part of the Life Bitch weight-loss programme. Don't give me a lame excuse that you can't spend ten minutes each day updating the journal that will take you through to Life Bitch success.

You should include the following sections daily in your life journey. Use the examples below as guidelines.

Motivation and willpower

✓ I bought a new pair of jeans two sizes smaller than my size now and hung them up next to my bedroom mirror.

✓ I arranged to take the kids ice-skating next month.

✓ The Christmas cake I've been nibbling at has gone in the bin.

✓ Carole asked me to go for a curry on Friday; I persuaded her to come round to me for a Life Bitch meal instead.

Self-affirmations

✓ I successfully avoided having a packet of crisps and some chocolate at work by picturing the sickness they would have caused in my body.

✓ In three weeks I'm going to ride the new bike I've bought with the kids. I picture this as I carry out my daily Life Bitch walks.

✓ I've binned the junk food that was in the house. It felt great, and now I'm not going into the fast-food joint where I normally pick up my lunch. I now picture 'slow food' and slow eating.

Food

✓ I've planned my first Life Bitch three-week menu. Tonight I ate baked salmon for the first time and I loved it.

✓ Instead of my usual Saturday fried breakfast at Sam's Café, I'm going to save the money and cook myself some grilled tomatoes, a bit of lean bacon and some mushrooms. I'm doing it for myself!

✓ I cancelled the weekly food delivery and wrote a healthy shopping list with the family. We are off to the supermarket later to buy food the Life Bitch way.

Exercise

✓ I went on my first Life Bitch walk. I felt achy afterwards because it's the first time I've moved my arse just for the sake of it in a long time, but I also feel fantastic about myself.

✓ I booked some tennis lessons for me and the kids next month, as it was something I did at college and really loved.

✓ I walked for 40 minutes today and took on the hill that always made me want to jump in the car on the way to Denise's house. I feel fantastic. I'm becoming a true Life Bitch!

✓ I'm fit and slim enough to start Pilates classes next week with a couple of mates. I can't wait.

The Life Bitch in me

✓ I told Sarah I didn't want to meet her for tea and cakes today, as I was going out on a walk. She said I was getting too obsessed with slimming and I told her she should join me at the park instead of the café. She's going to think about it. If she chooses to stay a fat-arsed baboon, that's her choice.

✓ I walked past the fish and chip shop yesterday evening and saw some real sights that couldn't even wait to get outside the shop before they stuffed the greasy chips and fatty batter down their gobs. It made me feel sick. I prefer fresh fish and vegetables these days. I'm beginning to notice the colours of the vegetables on my plate, and it reminds me that my personality is becoming more colourful as I lose weight. I am being eyed up more and more each day. I'm beginning to feel so sexy!

✓ The company's summer ball is six weeks away and I will have dropped at least one dress size, so I'm thinking of getting something really 'wow' to wear. I'm going to flirt with Peter from the sales department!

Life Bitch

Six good things

✓ I tried porridge for the first time this morning, with a tiny bit of honey. It tasted fab.

✓ I actually ran with the dogs on our walk today for the first time ever.

✓ I said 'no' to the Friday cakes in the office. Everyone was a bit stunned and my friend Sean said, 'You're so good!' I told myself, 'I know I am; I'm a Life Bitch winner!'

✓ Today I asked Matt to make a new hole in my belt, as it was too big.

✓ Last night I was out clubbing. I wore the short dress I'd dreamt of for ages and got chatted up more than once!

✓ My boss said I was really confident at the team meeting and that it was like I was someone else.

Six things to improve on

✓ I'm going to stop having butter on my toast in the mornings.

✓ The walks I go on will increase in intensity from Monday.

✓ I'm going to make homemade chips for the family tomorrow and throw away the frozen ones.

✓ I'm switching my self-motivation slot to 11 a.m., to make sure I don't get distracted by the kids.

✓ When I meet my friends tomorrow, I will ask one of them to be my Life Bitch buddy.

✓ I'm going to talk about my Life Bitch goals with the family — how they can help me and the rewards and incentives we should work together for. I'm going to buy tickets for Take That in June — that will get their attention.

The Life Bitch lifesavers

At times you will have doubts and face challenges that you feel threaten your position as a Life Bitch success. I want you to have this brief tool kit written up in the back of your journal to pull out when you need it. This is one of the lifesavers that will keep you true to the Life Bitch programme.

✗ Someone offers food you know you don't want, but you hesitate.

⬣ **Picture the big red stop sign.**

✗ You can't be arsed to get out of bed at the weekend to go for your daily walk.

⬣ **Take a look at the hideous picture of you and let that kick you up the backside.**

✗ You're at a wedding and you feel you've had too much champagne and now want to tuck into the wine.

⬣ **Head for the toilet, pull out your affirmations list and the gross picture and get a grip.**

Don't-panic menus and quick troughs

At the back of your journal, I want you to have a few quick-menu ideas that will keep you on the Life Bitch path. These are for when you simply don't have time to plan and you've got to put a meal together with no notice. I also want you to jot down some ideas for healthy snacks that will get you through when you think hunger is attacking. Go to pages 239–51 for menu ideas and pages 66–67 for quick-trough plans.

Goodies

Apricots

Asparagus

Avocado

Banana

Basil

Broccoli

Celery

Cottage cheese

Couscous

Crab

Eggs

Figs

Fresh fruit salad

Garlic

Grilled lean chicken

Lean steak

Lettuce

Life Bitch

Low-calorie bread

Low-fat mayonnaise

Mangetout

Pistachio nuts

Potatoes

Pumpkin

Salmon

Skimmed milk

Spinach

Squash

Strawberries

Sweet potatoes

Tofu

Tomatoes

Water

Wholegrain pasta

Yogurt

Baddies

Battered fish

Beef burgers

Butter

Chips

Chocolate biscuits

Cream

Cream cakes

Crisps

Doughnuts

Full-fat cheese

Full-fat fizzy drinks

Full-fat mayonnaise

Ice cream

Onion bhajis

Pasties

Pastry

Peanut butter

Life Bitch

Pints of beer

Pizza

Pork pie

Pork scratchings

Processed meat

Sausage rolls

Sherry

Steak pie

Sticky toffee pudding

Sweets

Toffee

Treacle

Index

Life Bitch

life BITCH!™

Watch out for more great titles from Steve Miller, coming soon from Headline Publishing Group, helping you make the changes – in areas ranging from your love life to your work life – that you want to make.

For more information about forthcoming Steve Miller events and publications, go to www.lifebitch.com